BOSH!

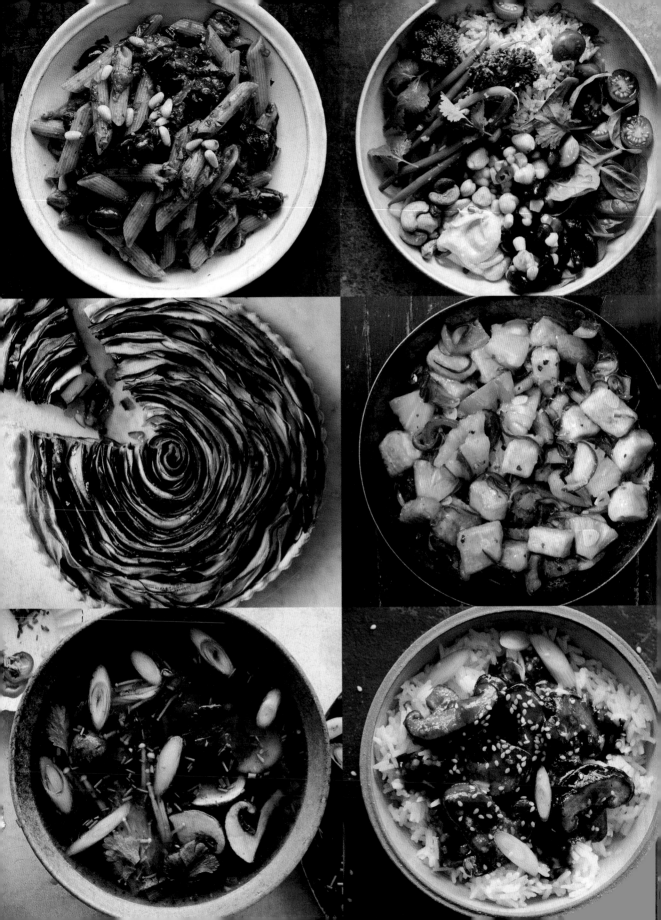

SIMPLE RECIPES
AMAZING FOOD
ALL PLANTS

BOSH!

This book is dedicated to you, whoever and whatever you are. We hope this book pleases and delights you, and takes you on a journey.

HarperCollins books may be purchased for educational, business, or sales promotional use. For information, please email the Special Markets Department at SPsales@harpercollins.com.

Originally published in the United Kingdom in 2018 by HQ, an imprint of HarperCollins Publishers.

FIRST U.S. EDITION

Photography: Lizzie Mayson

Food Styling: Pip Spence

Prop Styling: Sarah Birks

Design & Art Direction: Paul Palmer-Edwards, GradeDesign.com

Senior Commissioning Editor: Rachel Kenny

Project Editor: Sarah Hammond

Head of Design: Louise McGrory

Printed and bound in the USA

Library of Congress Cataloging-in-Publication Data has been applied for.

ISBN 978-0-06-282068-6

18 19 20 21 22   QVE   10 9 8 7 6 5 4 3 2 1

Contents

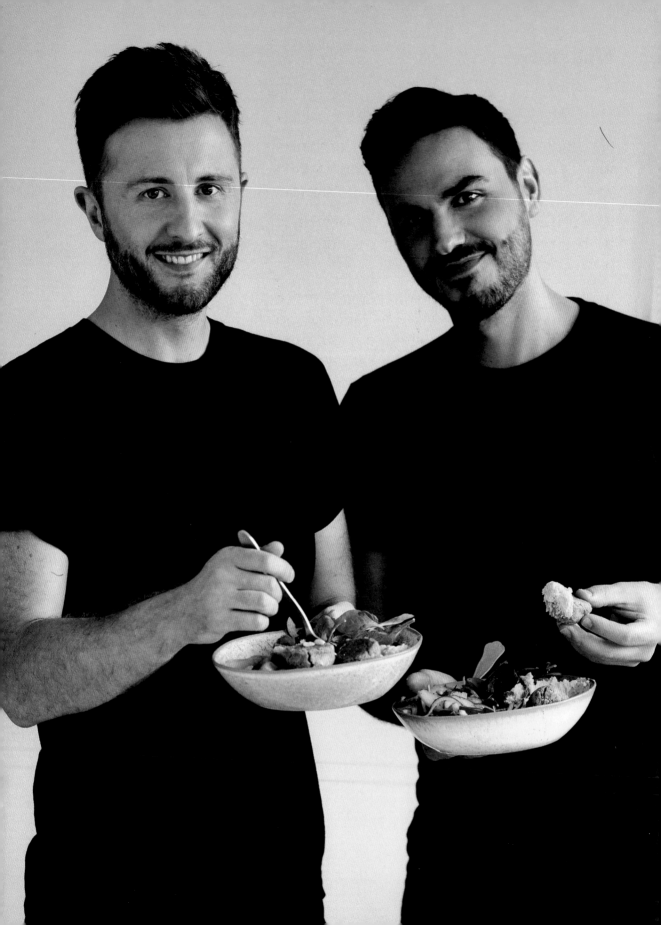

Welcome

We're here to show you how you can eat delightful meals that are both easy to cook and incredibly satisfying, all using just plants.

Let us introduce you to a new way of thinking about food; one that we've developed and perfected together over the last three years, and that is becoming increasingly popular.

It involves eating delicious, hearty, even indulgent meals that are both comfortingly familiar and exciting, and without any need for meat or dairy.

It's also a new way of cooking. Animal products are so ingrained in the human diet that we've had tens of thousands of years to hone the art of cooking with them. But the concept of cooking without meat and dairy is still relatively new. Which can only mean one thing: there is so much potential yet to be unleashed from plant-based eating.

We promise you'll find in this book your new, fail-safe family favorites, inspiring lunch ideas, showstoppers that'll impress even the most staunch steak-lover, tasty snacks, outrageously good desserts (we're pretty good at those, if we do say so ourselves), and awesome cocktails, every one bursting with flavor.

So, whether you're thinking about reducing the amount of meat you eat, or you don't eat animal products at all, this book is for you.

BOSH!

If you'd told us three years ago we were going to spend our lives cooking and eating amazing plant-based food, we wouldn't have believed you. We were a couple of mates from Sheffield who ate meat every single week.

Now we run BOSH!, the biggest plant-based online channel in the world. Our food creations were viewed by half a billion people in our first year and our most popular recipe videos have been viewed over 50 million times. We never expected to have that kind of success, and it has been humbling.

"I was the one to first cut out animal products."
Ian

"I mocked Ian when he went vegan, and asked him where he'd get his protein from. But eventually he won me over. That and the whole saving the world by not eating mass-produced animal products thing."
Henry

After cutting out animal products entirely, both of us felt fantastic. But we had to re-learn how to cook and find food when we were out and about. We also found that the vegan food available in restaurants or in cookbooks was often, frankly, not very good.

We saw an opportunity. Since then, it's been our life's mission to show people how to make delicious plant-based meals. However often they choose to do that.

And now, after three years of eating plant-based food, we've mastered a new style of cooking, one made popular through a new breed of internet chefs, where novelty and wow-factor presentation are just as important as taste and ease.

With this new style of cooking, we've created all-plants versions of classic dishes that are free from meat, eggs, and dairy, but still totally scrumptious. You know your favorite dishes, the ones you've learned by heart and use again and again? Well these are your new go-to classics.

Everything we do is aimed at showing just how easy it is to eat more plants. We also want to prove how delicious, hearty, and satisfying plant-based food can be.

We cook, drink, and film delicious recipes for the world, all from our home studio in East London.

x Henry and Ian

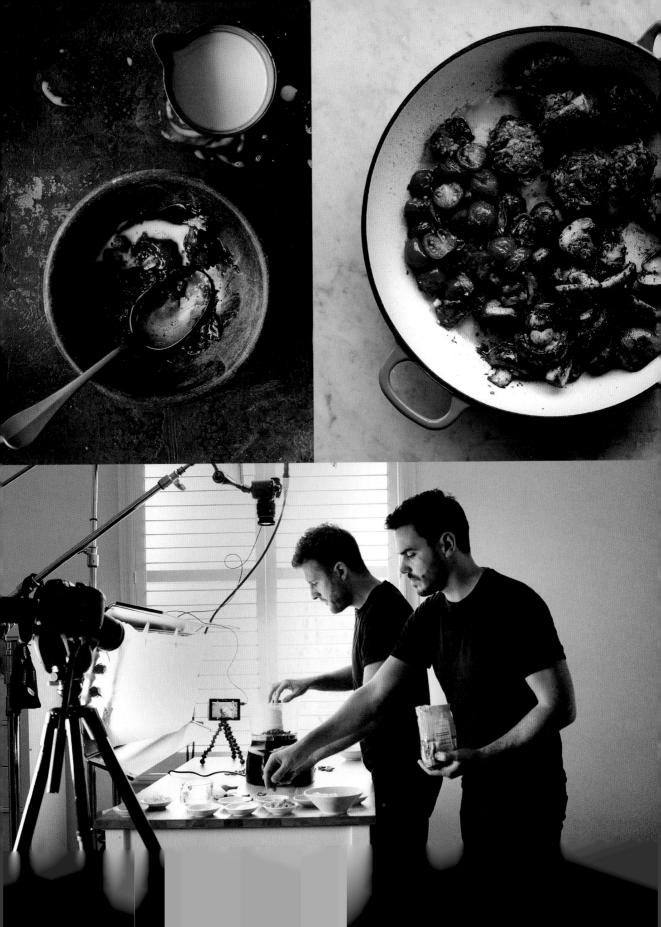

This book

Cook fast food fast. Spend time on showstoppers.
Sometimes you just need to eat quick, and you reach for your classic speedy dishes. Check out our Quick Eats chapter for yummy plates that you'll be able to get on the table in 30 minutes or less. Other times you're cooking for an occasion and looking to impress. Check out our Big Eats chapter for classics that will be worth the extra time, taking up to an hour to prep, or our Showpieces chapter for masterpieces that take that little bit longer (but the results are well worth it).

Get it right. First time. These are high-quality recipes.
Every recipe in this book has been rigorously and repeatedly tested again and again by us and our wonderful food team. We give you our word that these recipes work to a level that many in other cookbooks do not. These are high-quality recipes. Get the right tools, follow the instructions, and you can easily cook these meals to perfection.

To make it easier for you to work quickly, we've also included the preparation instructions (like peeling and chopping) in the method. This ensures that you make the best use of your time, cooking as quickly as possible. We've also included a "before you start" section above each recipe method, to highlight any special equipment you need or anything you should do before you start cooking. All oven temperatures are for convection ovens, so adjust the temperature if you have a conventional oven.

Create restaurant-quality meals at home
Check out our Fantastic Feasts section on page 17 to create menus as good as (or better than) anything you'll get from a restaurant or takeout, with dishes that complement each other.

Whether you're in the mood for an Asian blowout, an Indian banquet, a Tex-Mex spread, or a big Sunday lunch, you'll find everything you need in this book.

Watch videos to see how we do it
Looking for a helping hand when cooking a recipe? We've created a simple, top-down recipe video for the trickier dishes so you can see exactly how to cook them, step by step. Check out our website www.bosh.tv

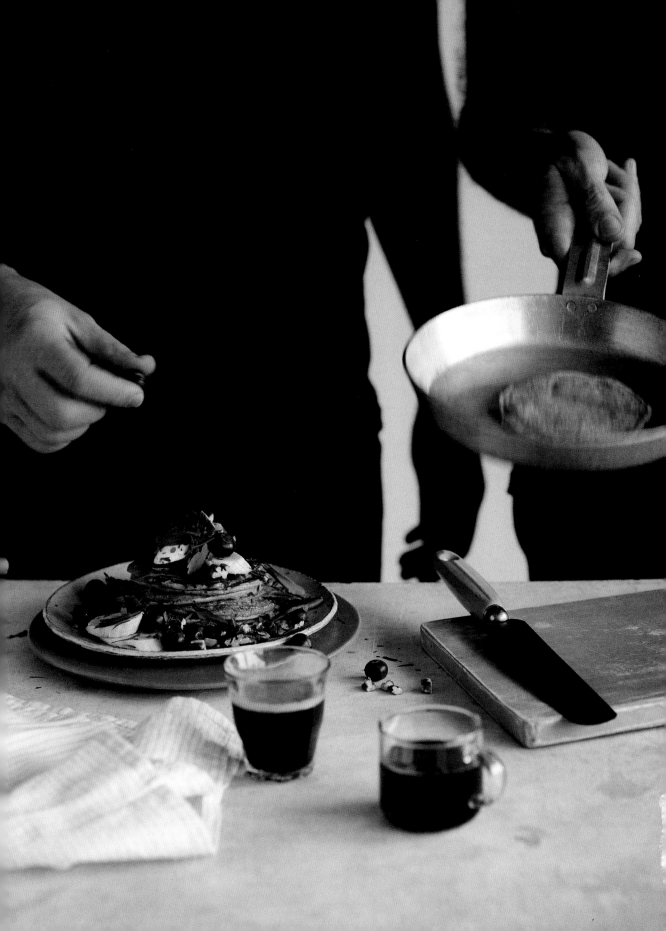

Your kitchen

Here are a few tips from us to help you really master your kitchen and your cooking skills.

Be a continuously improving cook, whatever your level
Whether you're just starting out cooking only with plants or you're already accomplished with vegan food, there's always something new to learn. Here's how to be at the top of your game.

Treat each recipe you cook as an opportunity to learn something new. Don't fall into the trap of cooking the same things on repeat; find new recipes, get the right ingredients, and try them out.

Up your skills from time to time with videos and books. Improve your knife skills with videos on YouTube. Use any of the amazing online tools, or a collection of cookbooks, to store up recipes to try in future. You can use post-its to mark the pages with recipes you want to try!

There's always something new to master, whether it's basics like getting vegan béchamel nailed or advanced baking with aquafaba. This new, plant-based way of thinking about food has so much freedom for innovation, so you'll be constantly improving.

Keep fruit and veggies on hand (or on ice) at all times!
A fridge full of fruit and veggies is not only good for your pocket, but they'll also keep really well. Onions, garlic, and potatoes are best kept out of the fridge in a cool, dry place.

Got lots of fruit left over? Stick it in the freezer and use it to make morning smoothies. Peel and chop the fruit into bite-sized chunks and put it into a Tupperware container for easy use later. We have a constant store of frozen bananas, apples, berries, spinach, kale, and watermelon ready to combine for a deliciously nutritious smoothie at any time of the day.

Bought too many veggies? That's OK: freeze them and use them later. Made too much pasta sauce? Pop it in a Tupperware or a freezer bag and keep it ready for a quick meal.

Keep your kitchen and pantry well organized to make life easier
Organize your pantry well and you'll always have meals ready to cook—check out page 15 for key ingredients to keep in stock. We go full nerd with sticky labels to highlight the right places for things. It makes cooking so much more satisfying and efficient because we're not constantly searching for ingredients in the cupboard.

We tend to organize our pantry shelves into sections like "sauces & syrups," "oils & vinegars," "herbs & spices," "flour, sugar & baking," "grains, rice, pasta," plus the essential "tea & coffee" shelf. Figure out a system that works for you. Trust us, knowing where things are makes fast cooking much easier.

Finally, organize your spices in a way that's easy to browse. We prefer smaller tubs of spices since they tend to be a consistent size and they usually have labels on the top. Plus, big bags of spice are harder to store and spices tend to go off if they're left on the shelf for too long. You'll soon discover which herbs and spices you get through quickly and which are worth buying in bulk—try decanting them into jars and adding your own labels on the lid.

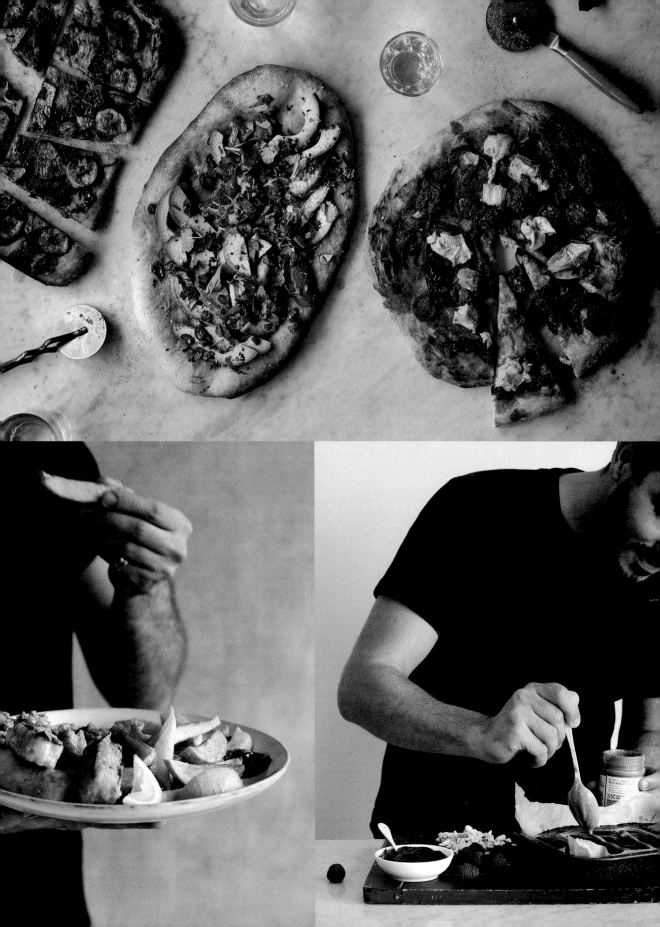

EQUIPMENT

The equipment you find in your typical kitchen is going to work just fine for the recipes in this book. There is nothing super fancy or technical about what we do in our kitchen; we like to keep things simple. But, if we were going to design a cost-effective kitchen from scratch, here's how we would do it:

Essential items

These should be your go-to items. We use these every day to make great BOSH! food.

High-powered blender (like a NutriBullet, Magic Ninja, or Magimix)

A **good, sharp knife** (and sharpener)

A selection of **cutting boards** that look great on the side and inspire you to cook

A **kitchen timer** or your mobile phone to get the timings right

Neatly stored spices, all in one place so you can find them quickly

A varied selection of preferably nonstick saucepans

Large spoons and tongs that work with your pans (don't use metal on nonstick!)

Measuring tools, like a measuring cup, scale, and measuring spoons

Nice-to-have items

Get these if you like. They will speed up your cooking, but they're optional.

Keep a clean **kitchen towel** in your pocket as you cook and you'll feel like a pro

Large-bowl **food processor** or **hand blender**

Oven-to-table dishes (for lasagna and pies)

Garlic crusher

A **grater** to zest or grate dairy-free cheese

A good **rolling pin**

Completely optional, but very cool items

These come in handy from time to time in our kitchen, so get them if you wish.

Pizza stone for better cooking and a crispier crust

Waffle iron

Toasted-sandwich maker

Slow cooker for long, slow, melt-in-the-mouth curries

Tiny dishes (soy sauce dishes) for measuring out spices before you start to cook

Sealing clips to keep opened packets of food from spilling everywhere

Tupperware or storage jars to keep your cupboards organized and store leftovers

Tofu press to make it even easier to cook with tofu

14

INGREDIENTS

The chances are that you already have most of these ingredients in your cupboard or your fridge. What we hope this book will do is unlock the potential in your pantry, and help you turn that humble can of chickpeas into the most awesome falafel, or transform your usual pasta dish into something you'd be proud to serve at a dinner party. Get stocked up!

Essentials

If someone were to ask us what we keep in our kitchen cupboards, this would be the answer. We use these ingredients all the time and always keep them on hand so that we can whip up a quick meal without having to go to the store first.

Pasta, in all its many forms, will answer your hunger prayers

Having **rice** in the cupboard means you'll always have something to eat

Noodles are a great base for speedy, nourishing, and satisfying meals

Olive or peanut oil, to use sparingly when frying or roasting

Sea salt and black pepper to season to perfection and bring your food to life

Garlic, because it's the best thing ever, used by nearly every cuisine in the world

Canned chickpeas give you the wonder beans with which you can make hummus and falafel, plus aquafaba, an incredibly useful substitute for egg and dairy in cooking

Various canned beans will ensure you get your protein whenever you need it

A supply of **canned tomatoes** means you always have a base for sauces

A selection of spices for essential flavor—never underestimate their power

Fresh fruit, veggies, and herbs because your mum told you to eat your greens and she was right

Nuts and seeds are fantastic for flavor, terrific for texture, and super, super healthy

Peanut butter will give you energy, texture, and flavor in abundance

Plant-based milk will crop up in our recipes again and again—we like almond milk best

Canned coconut milk will help you craft creamy curries

Specialties

We tend to have these in our cupboards too, but we use them less frequently.

Nutritional yeast provides a nutty, cheesy taste and is a great source of vitamin B12

Cashews can be soaked and blended for cream or cooked for a satisfying crunch

Passata or tomato puree will help your Italian dishes come to life

Kalamata olives add wonderful flavor and robust texture

Sun-dried tomatoes offer an incredible depth of flavor

Jarred roasted peppers are great blended up to add to a tomato sauce or soup

Dairy-free cheese will provide familiarity and texture

Firm tofu gives bite and texture, as well as all-important protein

Nori helps you get a fishy, salty flavor and can be used to wrap sushi rolls

Capers offer a really individual, salty flavor

Soy cream introduces lovely silky, creamy textures

Dairy-free ice cream should always be in the freezer because, well, movie night

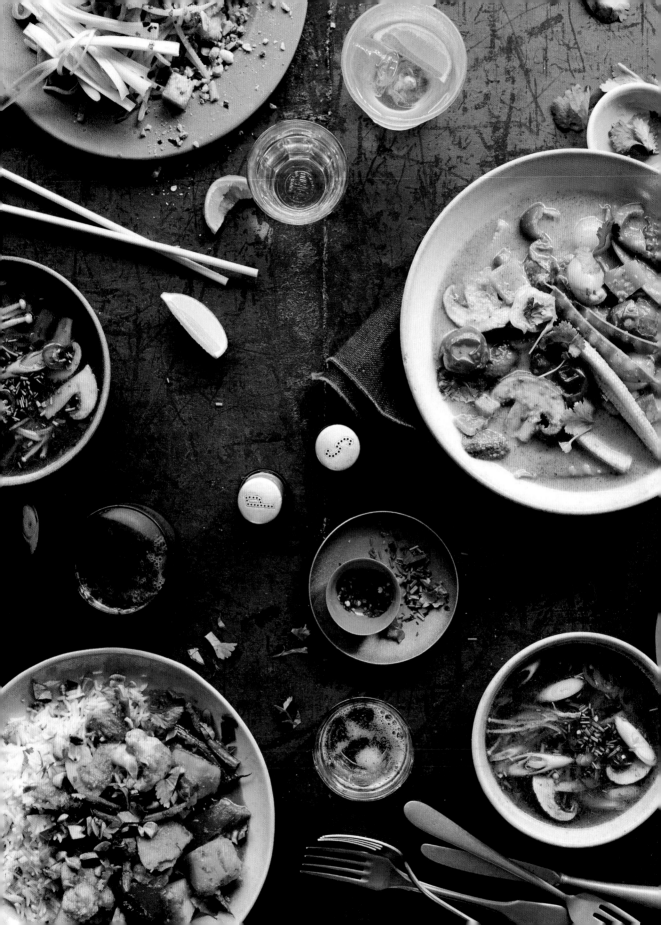

Fantastic feasts

Here are some delicious feasts you can create using the recipes in this book. Create your own takeout at home, or create a spread to wow a whole dinner party, using just this book.

SPANISH SPREAD

Fancy a fiesta? Make the ultimate Spanish spread. Just add sangria, salsa, and a little bit of sunshine.
Pettigrew's Paella (page 114)
Spanish Tapas (page 187)
Proper Spanish Aioli (page 192)

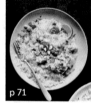
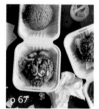
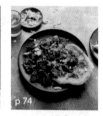

THE BIG INDIAN TAKEOUT

If contrasting curries is your thing then we've got you covered! This wonderful spread of curries, naan, and rice represents the best of our favorite cuisine.
Big Bhaji Burger (page 67)
Creamy Korma (page 71)
Rogan BOSH! (page 74)
Saag Aloo Curry (page 82)
Fluffy Naan Bread & Raita (page 203)
Onion Fried Rice (page 208)

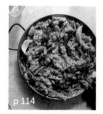
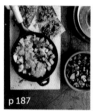
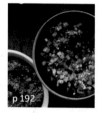
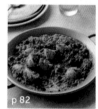
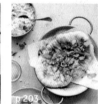
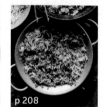

THE BIG THAI TAKEOUT

To magic up your own Southeast Asian takeout look no further than these recipes. You'll find deep, subtle yet strong spices and explosions of flavor.
Pad Thai (page 42)
Tom Yum Soup (page 63)
Thai Red Curry (page 78)
Massaman Curry (page 93)
(Rich Satay) Bangin' Veggie Kebabs (page 178)
Perfectly Boiled Rice (page 207)

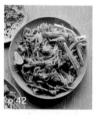
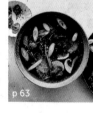
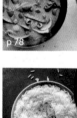
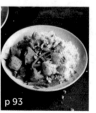
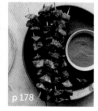
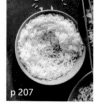

THE BIG CHINESE TAKEOUT

Create an Indo-Chinese takeout in your own home. Let your guests wrap their own pancakes, and pick and choose from all the bowls in the middle of the table. Just add chopsticks.

Sticky Shiitake Mushrooms (page 30)
Crispy Chili Tofu (page 46)
Sweet & Sour Crispy Tofu (page 59)
Shiitake Teriyaki Dippers (page 171)
Hoisin Pancakes (page 183)
Special Fried Rice (page 209)

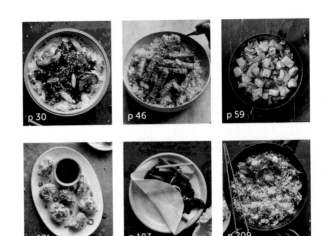

THE BIG BBQ

Feeling like an all-year-round taste of summer? These dishes will delight any BBQ party or brighten up any dining room. Grill and nibble to your heart's content.

Portobello Mushroom Burgers (page 45)
The Big BOSH! Burger (page 119)
Lemon & Chili Griddled Greens (page 147)
Ultimate BBQ Coleslaw (page 148)
Guacamole Potato Salad (page 151)
Bangin' Veggie Kebabs (page 178)

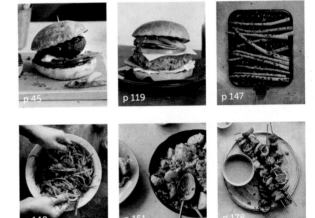

ITALIAN HEAVEN

If you like pasta and pizza as much as we do, then look no further. This is the perfect dinner-party spread.

Spaghetti Bolognese (page 86)
Perfect Pizza (page 107)
World's Best Pesto Lasagna (page 138)

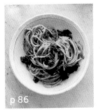
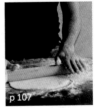
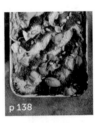

WEEKEND LUNCH

A British dinner of comfort and joy!

Mushroom & Guinness Pie (page 56)
"Fish" & Chips (page 134)
Sticky Toffee Pudding (page 245)

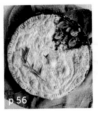
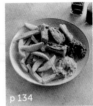
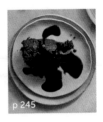

FANTASTIC FEASTS

A TEX-MEX-STYLE FIESTA

Combine these dishes for a serious taste of Tex-Mex goodness. We hope you like guacamole (who doesn't?). Feel free to dial down the chili if you prefer!

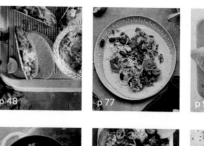
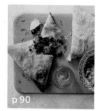
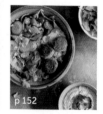
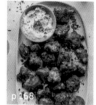

p 48 · p 77 · p 90

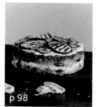
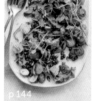
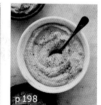

p 102 · p 103 · p 168

THE MEZZE PLATTER

Take a trip to the Middle East with the ultimate mezze spread. The flavors of hummus, falafel, and olives are deliciousness in every mouthful. If you have the time, trust us, the Mezze Cake is worth it.

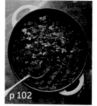
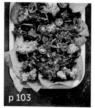
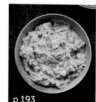

p 98 · p 144 · p 152

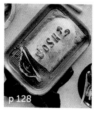
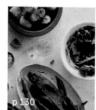
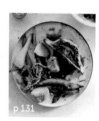

p 172 · p 193 · p 198

THE BIG BOSH! ROAST

No Sunday (or Christmas Day!) is complete without a roast dinner and all the trimmings. There are step-by-step instructions on page 127.

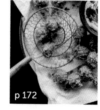

p 128 · p 130 · p 131

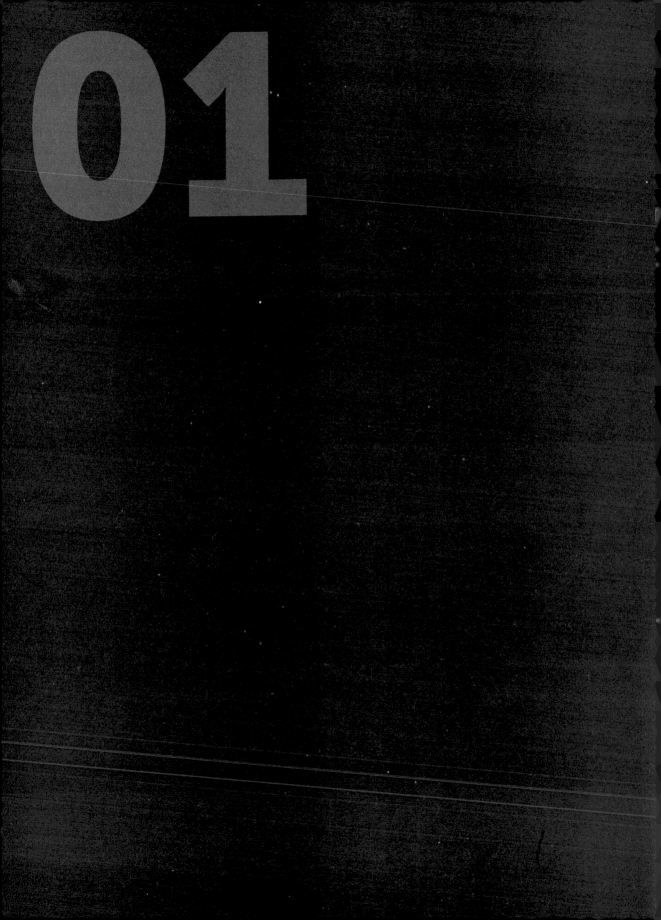

01

QUICK
EATS

Get it done quickly
Delicious food whenever
You need a fast feed

CREAMY CARBONARA

This is everything a carbonara should be: creamy, rich, and comforting. The smoky, flavorful mushrooms complement the thick, satisfying pasta sauce perfectly. A truly fantastic option for a delicious midweek dinner.

SERVES 4

6 portobello mushrooms (about 9 oz)
5 tbsp soy sauce
1 tbsp + 1 tsp maple syrup
1 tbsp + 1 tsp apple cider vinegar
1 tbsp + 1 tsp olive oil
4½ oz cashews
5 garlic cloves
generous ¾ cup unsweetened plant-based milk
2 tbsp nutritional yeast
5 oz silken tofu
10 oz spaghetti
1 cup green peas
handful flat-leaf parsley
   or arugula leaves, to serve

Preheat oven to 390°F | Line a baking sheet | Blender | Small saucepan of boiling water over high heat | Large saucepan of salted water over high heat

Slice the mushrooms thinly | Pour the soy sauce, maple syrup, cider vinegar, and olive oil into a bowl and whisk to combine | Add the mushrooms, making sure the slices are well covered in the marinade, and set aside

Meanwhile, put the cashews in the small saucepan filled with boiling water and boil for 15 minutes

Take the mushroom slices out of the bowl and lay them out evenly on the lined baking sheet | Add the whole garlic cloves and pour the marinade over everything | Bake in the hot oven for 25–30 minutes, until they have shrunk in size and begun to crisp very slightly

Drain the cashews and put them into the blender along with the plant-based milk, nutritional yeast, and tofu | Whizz to a very smooth cream and then set aside

Add the pasta to the large pan of boiling salted water and cook until al dente, following the instructions on the packet | Add the peas for the last minute of cooking | Fill a mug with pasta water and set aside | Drain the pasta and peas in a colander and tip the pasta back into the cooking pot

Pour the carbonara cream and 3 tablespoons of the pasta water over the pasta and stir everything around until the pasta is well covered in the cream | Take the mushrooms out of the oven and fold them into the creamy pasta | Add another splash of pasta water, if needed, to give a nice, loose, creamy consistency

Garnish with the fresh parsley or arugula (or any other leafy green) and serve immediately

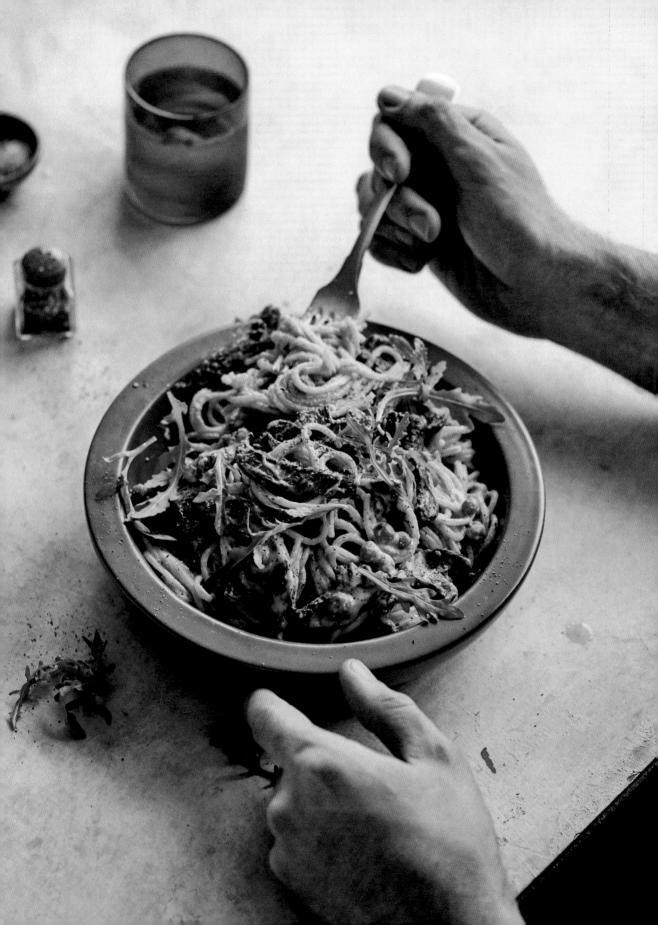

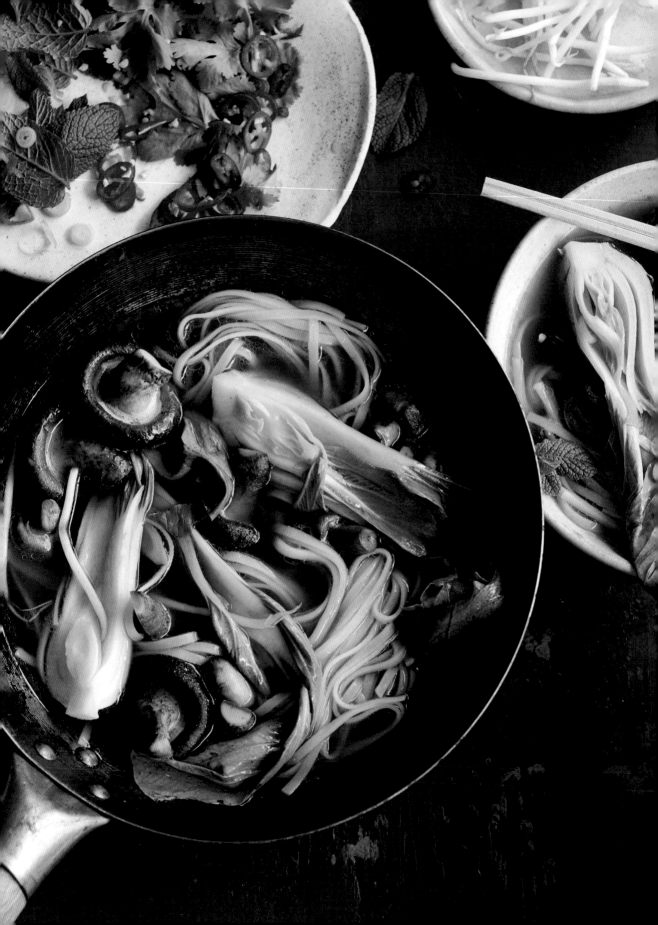

MUSHROOM PHO

Nothing beats a hearty pho soup. Traditionally, pho is made with a deep stock that's been brewing for hours, or even days. We've used a shortcut but retained the pho richness through the delights of shiitake mushrooms, star anise, and tamarind paste. Just make sure you have enough liquid and add more water if you need to.

SERVES 6

2 onions
4 garlic cloves
3-inch piece fresh ginger
3 fresh red chilies
16 shiitake mushrooms
6 tbsp toasted sesame oil
⅔ cup fresh orange juice
   (not from concentrate)
2 tbsp tamarind paste
4 star anise
2 cinnamon sticks
3 quarts water
7 tbsp soy or tamari sauce
7 tbsp maple syrup
10 button mushrooms
10 oz flat rice noodles
4 scallions
2 handfuls fresh cilantro
2 handfuls fresh mint
5 oz bean sprouts
7 oz bok choy
sriracha and soy sauce, to serve

Large saucepan over medium heat

Peel and coarsely chop the onions and garlic | Peel the ginger by scraping off the skin with a spoon and chop coarsely | Rip the stem from one of the chilies and chop, removing the seeds if you prefer a milder flavor | Trim and roughly slice 6 of the shiitake mushrooms

Heat 3 tablespoons of the sesame oil in the large saucepan and add the chopped onion, garlic, chili, ginger, and the sliced shiitakes | Cook for 10–15 minutes, stirring continuously until everything has softened

Add the orange juice, tamarind paste, star anise, and cinnamon sticks and continue to stir for another 3 minutes | Add the water, soy, or tamari sauce and maple syrup

Turn up the heat, bring to a boil, then turn it down again and simmer for 10 minutes, until reduced by about one-sixth | Strain the liquid into a large bowl through a sieve | Rinse the pan

Put the pan back over high heat and add the remaining 3 tablespoons sesame oil | While the oil is warming, trim the remaining 10 shiitakes and the button mushrooms and add them to the pan | Fry for a couple of minutes, until very slightly browned | Pour all the pho liquid back into the pan | Add the rice noodles and cook for about 3–4 minutes, or according to the package directions

Finely slice the scallions and put them in a small pile on a large plate | Pick the leaves from the cilantro and mint and put them on the plate | Trim and finely slice the remaining chilies, removing the seeds if you prefer a milder flavor, and put them on the plate along with the bean sprouts

Trim and quarter the bok choy lengthwise and add it to the soup | Take the whole pan to the table along with the plate, with a ladle for people to serve themselves and chopsticks for them to add their own fresh herbs, vegetables, and chilies | Serve with soy sauce and sriracha on the side | Best eaten as soon as it's ready!

GUACARONI

Macaroni meets guacamole! This dish is as perfect as its name suggests and we think it's one of the finest pasta salads you will ever taste. It's great eaten hot or cold, served alongside a BBQ, as a lunchtime salad, or with a bit of green salad as a quick main course.

SERVES 4–6

11 oz macaroni
3½ tsp salt
4 ripe avocados
2 limes
2 tbsp olive oil
½ tsp garlic powder
½ red onion
2 fresh red chilies
12 cherry tomatoes
1 cup fresh cilantro leaves

Large saucepan of water over high heat | Large mixing bowl

Add the macaroni and 2 teaspoons of the salt to the boiling water and cook until al dente, according to the package directions

Halve and carefully pit the avocados by tapping the pits firmly with the heel of a knife so that it lodges in the pit, then twist and remove the pits, then scoop the flesh into the mixing bowl | Halve the limes and squeeze the juice into the bowl, catching any seeds in your other hand | Add the olive oil, garlic powder, and the remaining salt to taste and mash the avocado using the back of a fork | Peel and mince the onion | Rip the stems from the chilies, cut them in half lengthwise, and remove the seeds if you prefer a milder flavor | Finely chop the tomatoes, chilies, and cilantro and add to the bowl | Mix all the ingredients together

Drain the macaroni and tip into the bowl of guacamole, stirring to make sure the pasta is well covered | Serve immediately as a side dish or light lunch, or box it up ready for tomorrow's lunch

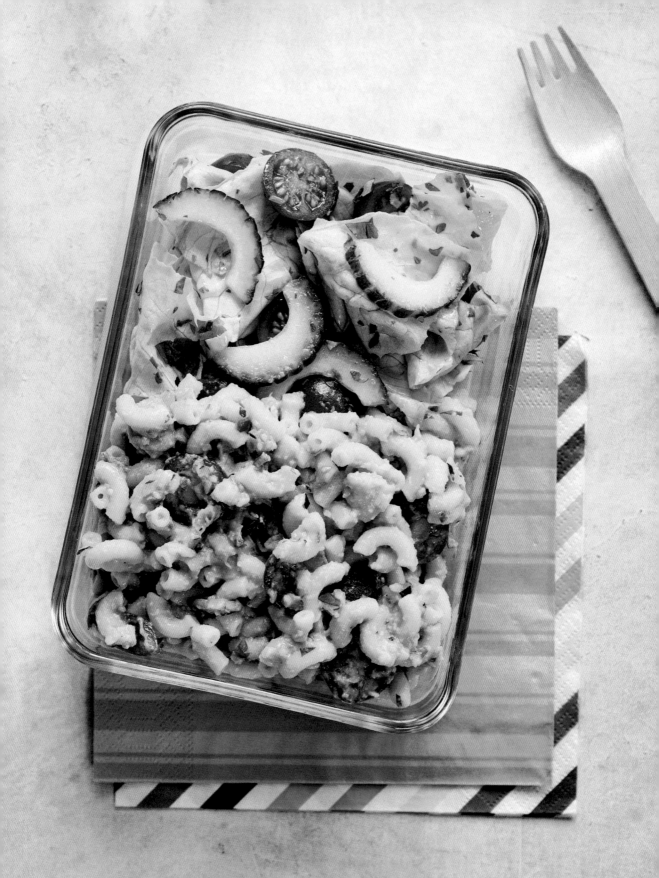

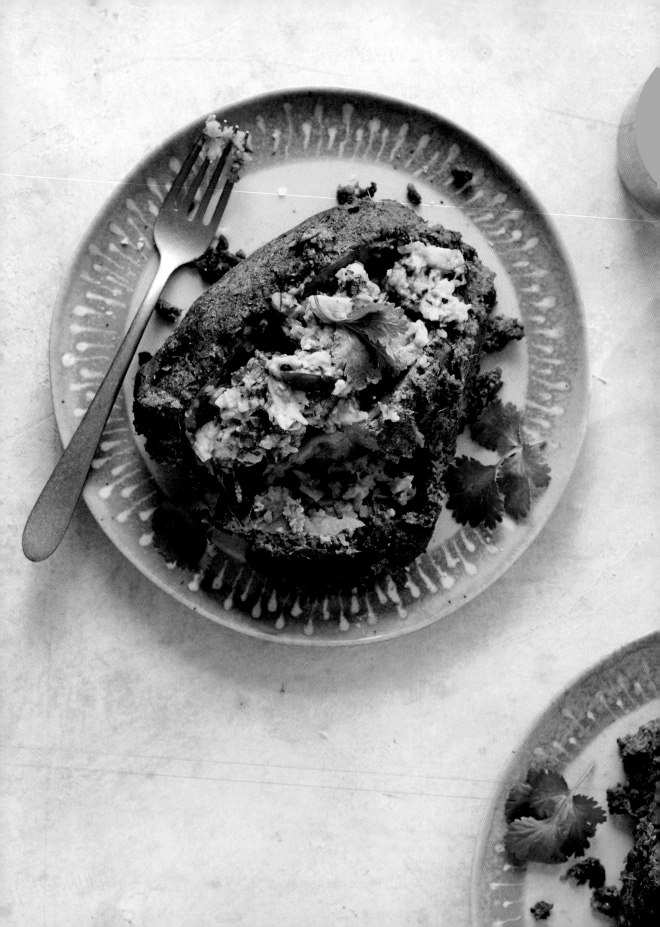

CURRY-CRUSTED SWEET POTATOES

We've mixed up the traditional stuffed potato by putting our filling on the outside in this recipe. The flavors work a treat with a fresh lime crust contrasting really well with a delicious sweet potato. This is one to freestyle with and try different flavor combos. It works great in the oven or cooked on an outdoor grill.

SERVES 2

2 large sweet potatoes
    (about 10 oz each)
vegetable oil, for greasing
salad leaves, to serve, optional
2 cups guacamole (store-bought
    or see page 194), to serve, optional

FOR THE CURRY PASTE
2-inch piece fresh ginger
3 garlic cloves
1 fresh red chili
1 lime
8 sun-dried tomatoes,
    plus 1 tbsp oil from the jar
15 sprigs fresh cilantro
7 tbsp shredded coconut
generous 1 tbsp panko breadcrumbs
1½ tsp salt
1 tsp garam masala
1 tsp ground cumin
2 tsp water

Preheat oven to 390°F | Food processor | Baking sheet | Foil

Prick the whole sweet potatoes with a fork and put them on a plate | Microwave on high for about 10–15 minutes until quite soft (alternatively put the potatoes in a 425°F oven and bake for 25 minutes, remove them from the oven, and reduce the heat to 390°F) | Remove and set aside to cool down slightly | Score the skins with a sharp knife

Peel the ginger by scraping off the skin with a spoon | Peel the garlic | Rip the stem from the chili, cut it in half lengthwise, and remove the seeds if you prefer a milder flavor | Cut the lime in half and squeeze the juice into the food processor, catching any seeds in your other hand | Put all the rest of the curry paste ingredients into the food processor and whizz to a thick paste

Cut 2 squares of foil big enough to fully wrap your sweet potatoes in and grease one side with oil | Take half the curry paste and use your hands to encase one of the potatoes with a thick layer of paste | Repeat with the second potato

Tightly wrap the sweet potatoes in the foil squares, put on the baking sheet, and bake in the preheated oven for 30 minutes | Take the sweet potatoes out of the oven, remove the foil, and serve with a small side salad and a big spoonful of guacamole, if using

STICKY SHIITAKE MUSHROOMS

If you're a fan of sticky, sweet, pan-Asian cuisine you will love this dish (seriously, it's bangin'!). It's quick and easy to put together and guaranteed to impress. Serve with freshly cooked rice and chopsticks.

SERVES 2

½ lb shiitake mushrooms
3 tbsp cornstarch
2 tbsp peanut oil
2 garlic cloves
1¼-inch piece fresh ginger
½ tsp water
1 tbsp toasted sesame oil
2 tbsp light brown sugar
¼ cup dark soy sauce
2 tbsp rice vinegar
1 tsp sriracha sauce, or to taste
1 scallion, to serve
2 cups cooked basmati rice
   (store-bought or Perfectly Boiled
   Rice, see page 207), to serve
1 tsp sesame seeds, to serve

Wok or large frying pan over high heat

Thickly slice the mushrooms and put them in a bowl | Sprinkle 2 tablespoons of the cornstarch over the top and toss everything together with your hands, making sure the mushrooms are well covered | Pour the peanut oil into the wok or pan and get it nice and hot | Tip in the mushrooms and fry for 4–6 minutes, until cooked through and slightly crisp on the outside | Transfer the mushrooms to a bowl and set aside

Peel and finely chop the garlic and ginger | Spoon the remaining 1 tablespoon cornstarch into a small dish and mix it together with the water | Wipe out the wok with paper towels and put it back over low heat | Pour in the sesame oil | Add the chopped garlic and ginger and cook until you release the aromas and they're bubbling in the oil, about 1 minute | Sprinkle in the sugar and stir until caramelized, about 2 minutes more | Increase the heat slightly and pour in the cornstarch mixture, soy sauce, and rice vinegar, then stir for another minute until the sauce has thickened slightly | Add the sriracha and stir it into the sauce | Tip the cooked mushrooms back into the pan and stir to warm through and completely cover in the sauce, 1–2 minutes longer

Finely slice the scallion | Serve the chewy mushrooms over hot basmati rice, garnished with the sliced scallion and sprinkled with sesame seeds

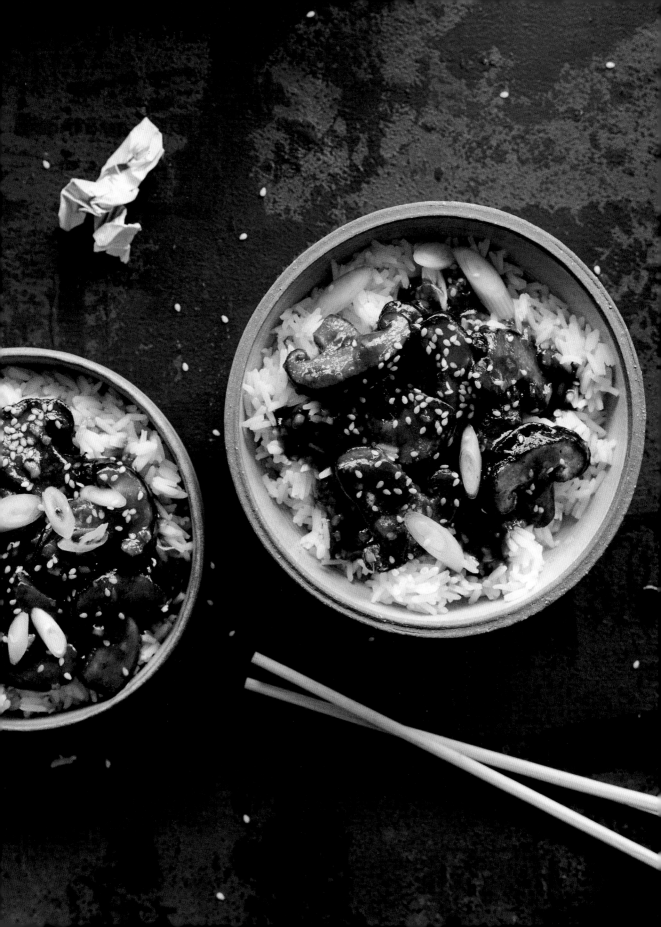

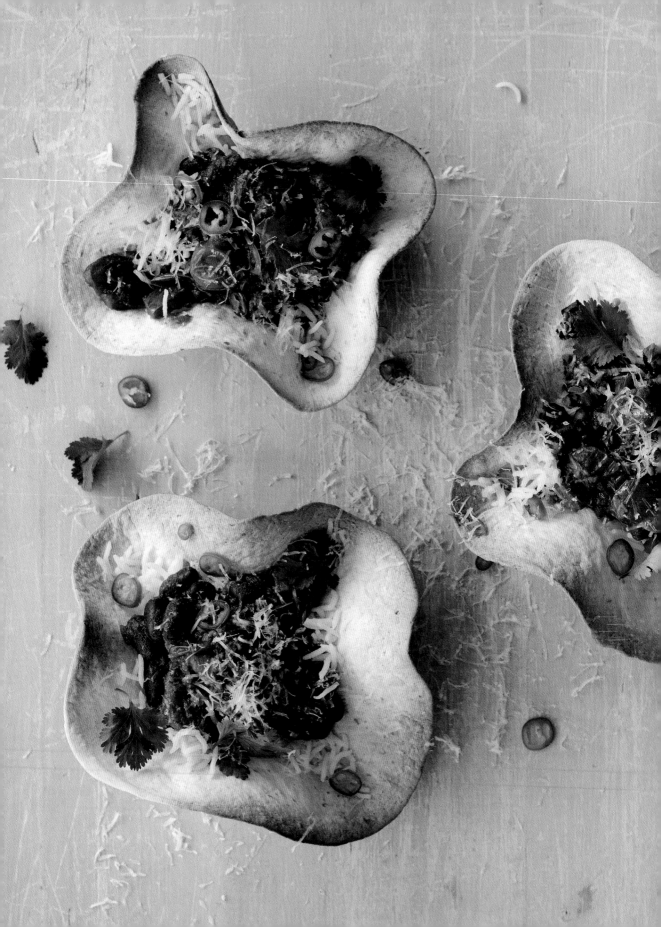

MINI CHILI BOWLS

This is a quick-to-prepare, warming hug-in-a-bowl kind of dish that's good for impressing your guests when time is against you! Feel free to up the chili if you like a bit of a kick. This banging chili is served inside a cool cone dish.

SERVES 3–6

3–6 medium flour tortillas
1 fresh red chili
1 red onion
2 garlic cloves
2 red bell peppers
9 sprigs fresh cilantro
12 cherry tomatoes
2 tbsp olive oil
1 tsp paprika
½ tsp ground cumin
1 can (15 oz) kidney beans
1 can (15 oz) black beans
24 oz tomato puree
3 cups cooked rice (store-bought or
   Perfectly Boiled Rice, see page 207)
1¾ oz dairy-free cheese, optional
1 lime

Preheat oven to 350°F | Muffin or cupcake tin | Lidded casserole or saucepan over medium heat

Turn the muffin or cupcake tin upside down and place 3 tortillas in the gaps between the cups, making 3 bowl shapes | Press each tortilla down firmly to get a flat bottom, to ensure the bowls will stand up | Place the tin in the oven and bake for 7–10 minutes until lightly browned and firm | Take out of the oven and leave to cool and harden on the tin | If you are cooking for more than 3 people, repeat this step with more tortillas

Rip the stem from the chili, cut it in half lengthwise, and remove the seeds if you prefer a milder flavor, then chop | Peel and chop the onion and garlic | Cut the bell peppers in half and cut out the stems and seeds, then chop | Cut the stems from the cilantro and finely chop, reserving the leaves for later | Halve the cherry tomatoes

Heat the olive oil in the pan and add the chopped chili, onion, garlic, and cilantro stems and cook for 5 minutes, stirring occasionally | Add the cherry tomatoes and bell peppers and stir for another 4–5 minutes | Add the paprika and ground cumin | Drain the kidney beans and black beans and stir into the sauce | Pour in the tomato puree | Leave the sauce to simmer for 10 minutes, stirring occasionally

Heat the rice, according to the package directions | Put a small layer of rice on the bottom of each of the tortilla bowls and top with a generous serving of chili | Grate the dairy-free cheese, if using, on top and sprinkle with the cilantro leaves | Cut the lime into wedges and place one on each plate to serve

QUICK PUTTANESCA SPAGHETTI

The combination of lemon and fresh parsley in this dish creates a voluptuous pasta and the saltiness of the capers in brine will remind you of the sea. This flexible favorite of ours is great for when you're low on fresh ingredients. It can be served with a side salad or makes a great quick meal all on its own.

SERVES 6

2 small red chilies, fresh or dried
20 sprigs flat-leaf parsley
10 Kalamata olives
4 garlic cloves
¼ cup olive oil
1 tbsp capers, plus 1 tbsp
   of brine from the jar
½ tsp salt, plus a little extra
24 oz tomato puree
1 lb spaghetti
½ lb broccolini
1 lemon

Large saucepan over medium-high heat | Large saucepan of boiling salted water over high heat

Rip the stems from the chilies, cut them in half lengthwise, and remove the seeds if you prefer a milder sauce, and finely chop | Separate the parsley stems and finely chop, reserving the leaves for later | Pit and roughly chop the olives

Peel 2 of the garlic cloves | Pour 2 tablespoons of the oil into the empty saucepan, crush in the garlic, and add the chilies, parsley stems, olives, and capers and stir for 2–3 minutes | Add the ½ teaspoon salt and 1 tablespoon of the salty brine water from the jar of capers | Leave to cook for a minute, then add the tomato puree | Taste and season with salt if necessary | Turn the heat to medium and leave to simmer while you move on to the next step

Add the spaghetti to the pan of boiling water along with the remaining 2 garlic cloves | Cook until al dente, according to the package directions

Meanwhile, carefully slice the broccolini from top to bottom, creating thin strips | Add these to the spaghetti pan for the last 30 seconds of cooking time to quickly soften | Drain the pasta and broccoli in a colander and return them to the pan | Pour in the sauce

Roughly chop the parsley leaves and add them to the pan | Pour in the remaining 2 tablespoons of oil and squeeze over the juice of a whole lemon, catching any seeds in your other hand | Mix everything together and serve immediately

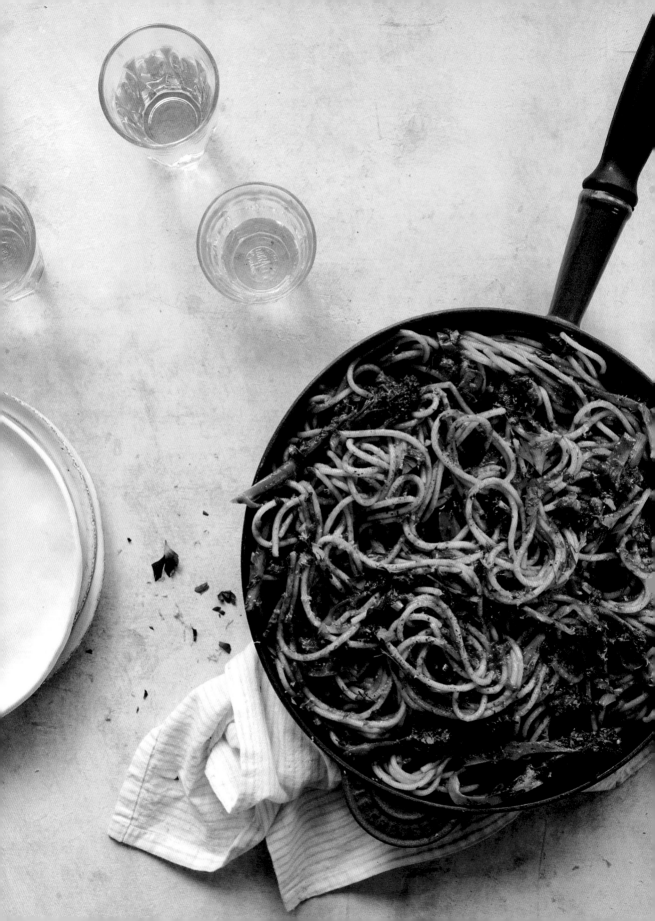

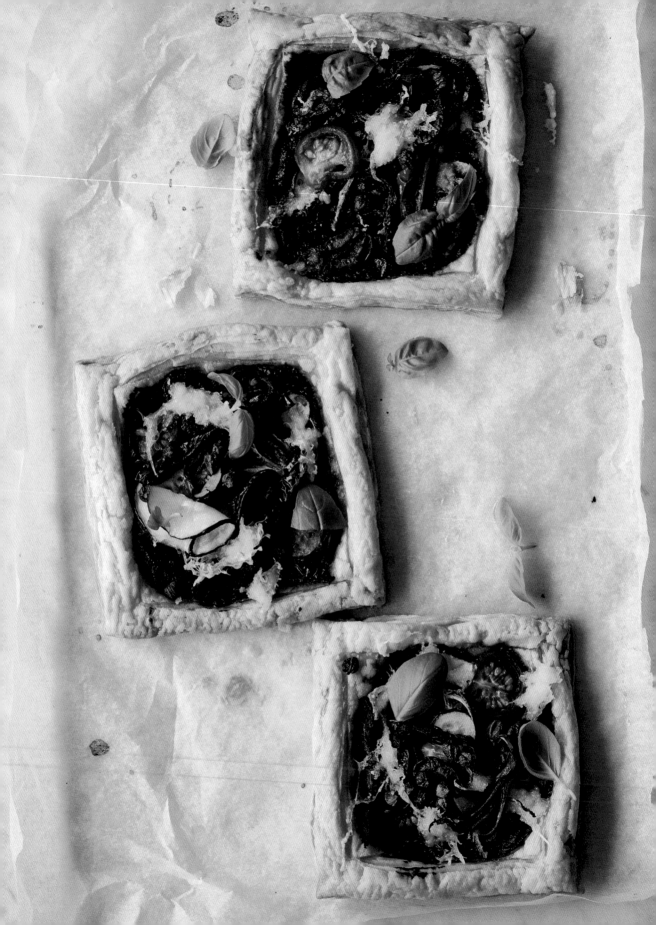

MINI PIZZA TARTS

These tarts are incredibly easy to prepare, really flavorful and look impressive. They're perfect for a starter or light lunch and are an opportunity for you to get creative with your decoration. The fluffy melt-in-your-mouth crunch of the pastry makes for a decadent but messy meal!

SERVES 6

1 sheet (11 oz) ready-to-bake dairy-free
    puff pastry
½ red onion
½ zucchini
12 cherry tomatoes
6 sun-dried tomatoes
2 tbsp capers
12 pitted Kalamata olives
2 tbsp unsweetened plant-based milk
1¾ oz dairy-free cheese, optional
handful small fresh basil leaves, to serve

FOR THE TOMATO SAUCE
3 tbsp tomato paste
1 tbsp olive oil
1 tbsp water
2 tsp balsamic vinegar
½ tsp black pepper
½ tsp salt

Preheat oven to 350°F | Baking sheet | Pastry brush

Unroll the puff pastry onto the baking sheet, keeping it on the parchment paper it's wrapped in | Take a sharp knife and cut the pastry into 6 equal squares and separate them slightly | Run the tip of the knife lightly around the edge of each square to score a ½-inch border

Put all the ingredients for the tomato sauce into a small bowl and mix with a fork | Spread the sauce inside each pastry square, up to the border

Peel the red onion and trim the zucchini and cherry tomatoes | Finely slice them along with the sun-dried tomatoes, capers and olives (it's important they be cut very fine so they cook quickly) | Arrange artfully over each pizza square, keeping the borders free | Brush the edges of the pizzas with the plant-based milk

Put the baking sheet in the oven and bake for 20–22 minutes, then remove and neatly grate the dairy-free cheese, if using, over the top of each square | Put the tarts back in the oven for 3 minutes to melt (if you cook them for any longer the cheese will start to harden)

Remove the pan from the oven, scatter the basil leaves over the tartlets and serve immediately

NICE SPICE RICE

This quick and easy dish is a regular late-night meal in the BOSH! studio. It's healthy, colorful, and also delicious, with a salty, sweet, nutty flavor and an incredible number of healthy veg. Works great as a quick meal or a side, or as a leftover lunch the following day!

SERVES 3—4

4 oz kale
9 sprigs fresh cilantro
2 large garlic cloves
2-inch piece fresh ginger
1 large fresh red chili
5 scallions
1 red bell pepper
1 tbsp coconut oil
1 tbsp toasted sesame oil
5 tsp maple syrup
¼ cup light soy sauce
3 oz baby corn
2 oz thin pencil asparagus spears
3 oz sugar snap peas
3 oz broccolini
scant ½ cup smooth peanut butter
2 tbsp water
4 cups cooked basmati rice
    (store-bought or homemade)
sriracha sauce, to serve, optional
fresh lime, to serve, optional
salt

Wok over medium heat

Chop the kale and cilantro and set aside | Peel and finely slice the garlic | Peel the ginger by scraping off the skin with a spoon and finely slice | Rip the stem from the chili, then cut it in half lengthwise and remove the seeds if you prefer a milder flavor | Finely chop the chili and scallions | Cut the bell pepper in half and cut out the stem and seeds, then cut into bite-sized chunks along with the rest of the vegetables | Measure out the oils, syrup, and soy sauce into saucers or small bowls ready to use

Add the coconut oil to the wok and stir until melted | Add the toasted sesame oil and let it infuse into the coconut oil | Add the garlic and ginger and stir them around for 1–2 minutes, until the ginger looks like it's begun to froth

Add the chopped chili and scallions and stir until the onions have softened | Pour in the maple syrup and soy sauce and stir | Add the corn, asparagus, and bell pepper and stir for roughly 1 minute | Throw in the sugar snap peas and broccolini and stir for another minute | Add the peanut butter and water to the pan and stir until all the vegetables are well covered | Finally, add the kale and stir until it is slightly wilted | Taste and season with salt if necessary | Turn the heat down to low

Add the rice to the wok and fold it into the vegetables for 2 minutes | Sprinkle with the cilantro and stir briefly to combine | Serve immediately with wedges of fresh lime and sriracha sauce on the side, if using

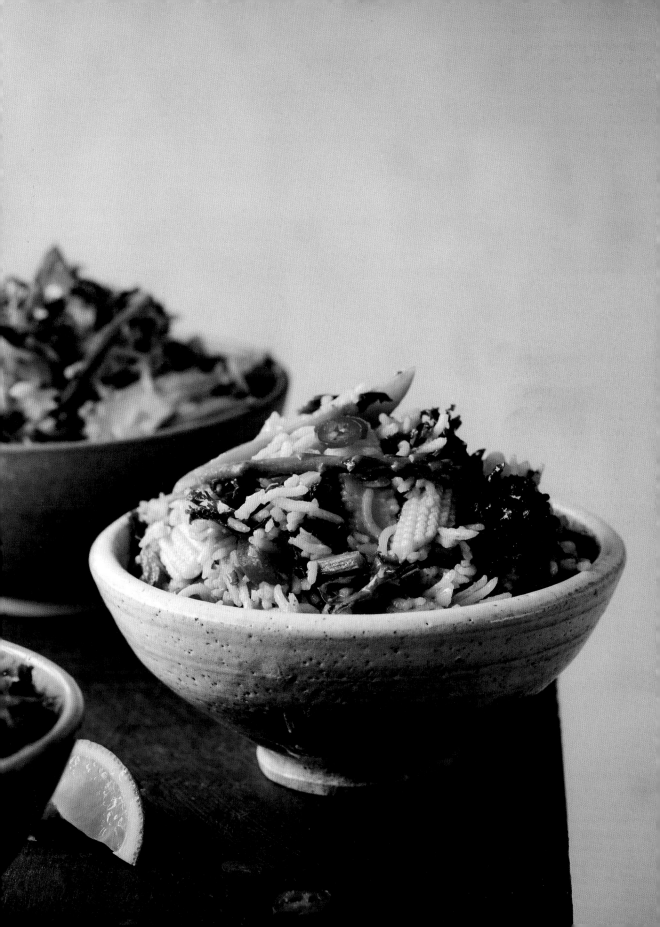

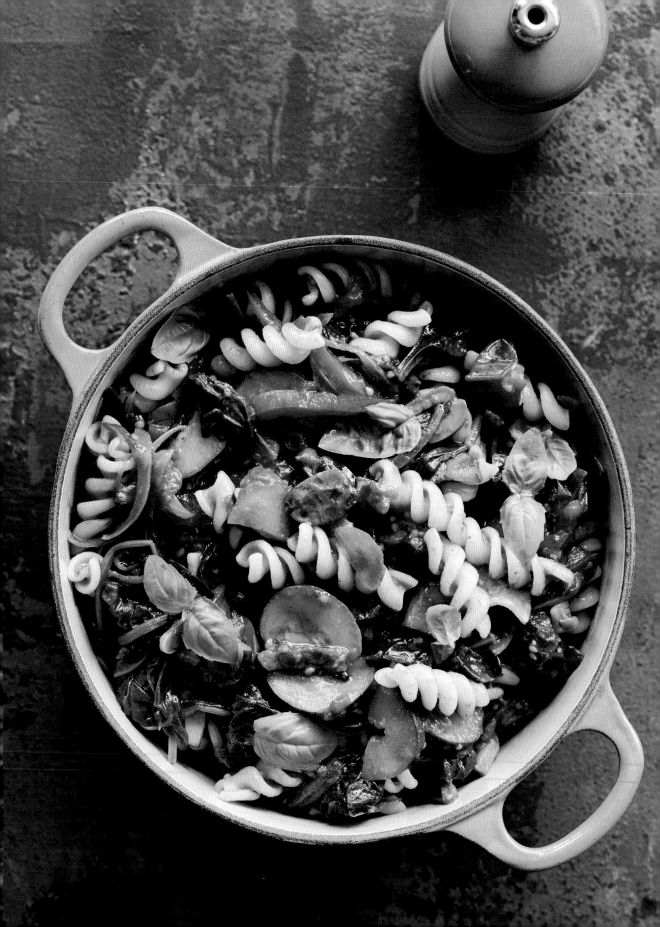

EASY PEASY PASTA

The clue is in the name with this one. It's an effortlessly simple pasta sauce that can be made with minimal effort, since it's mainly just roasted vegetables. It's a regular supper at BOSH! HQ. It's fresh, filling, and gives you loads of your daily vegetables in one lavish meal. Try serving it up with a side salad and some crusty bread.

SERVES 4

2 red onions
4 garlic cloves
2 red bell peppers
3½ oz sun-dried tomatoes
1½ oz baby spinach
4 tbsp capers
2 small zucchini
3½ oz pitted Kalamata olives
1 lb cherry tomatoes
½ cup oil (ideally from the
  sun-dried tomato jar!)
1⅓ cups tomato puree
11 oz fusilli
generous 1 cup basil leaves
salt and black pepper

Preheat oven to 350°F | 9 x 13-inch baking dish | Large saucepan

Peel and finely slice the onions and garlic | Cut the bell peppers in half, cut out the stems and seeds, and slice into thin strips | Slice the sun-dried tomatoes | Finely chop the spinach leaves and capers and chop the zucchini into bite-sized chunks | Halve the olives and tomatoes | Put all the vegetables into the baking dish and season all over with salt and pepper | Pour in the oil and tomato puree and stir to ensure all the vegetables are covered | Cover the dish with foil and put it in the oven to roast for 30 minutes

Take the dish out of the oven, remove the foil, stir everything, and put the dish back in the oven for 15 minutes longer

Meanwhile, bring a large pan of water to a boil over high heat | Add the pasta and a big pinch of salt and cook until al dente, according to the package directions | Drain the cooked pasta in a colander and tip it back into the pan

Take the baking dish out of the oven, stir in the basil leaves, and pour your freshly roasted veggie sauce over the pasta | Stir so that it's well mixed, serve and enjoy!

PAD THAI

In Thailand, pad Thai was a regular lunch for us (and the perfect remedy for a Thai-bucket-induced hangover). It varies everywhere you go, but typically includes the artful placement of fresh lime, peanuts, and scallions around the bowl. We like to replicate this and serve it with chili flakes, Thai sweet chili sauce, and sriracha.

SERVES 4

5 oz extra-firm tofu
1 tbsp cornstarch
¼ cup vegetable oil
7 oz flat dried rice noodles
½ onion
2 garlic cloves
1 fresh red chili
1 carrot
splash of water
3½ oz bean sprouts
3 limes
¼ cup soy sauce
2 scallions
½ cup unsalted peanuts
1 tbsp chili flakes, to serve
Thai sweet chili sauce, to serve, optional
sriracha sauce, to serve, optional

FOR THE DRESSING
1 tbsp palm sugar (or any sugar)
2 tbsp tamarind paste
1 tbsp sweet chili sauce

Tofu press or 2 clean kitchen towels and a weight such as a heavy book | Wok

Press the tofu using a tofu press or place it between two clean kitchen towels, lay it on a plate, and put a weight on top | Leave for at least 30 minutes to drain any liquid and firm up before you start cooking

In a bowl, mix together all the ingredients for the dressing

Take half the tofu and cut it into ⅓-inch cubes (save the other half for another time) | Sift over the cornstarch and turn the tofu to coat all over

Put the wok over high heat and pour in 2 tablespoons of oil | Add the tofu and immediately reduce the heat to medium | Stir gently, without breaking up the tofu, until lightly browned | Transfer to a plate

Bring water to a boil | Put the noodles in a bowl, cover them with the hot water, and leave for about 3 minutes, until they're flexible but not cooked (check the package directions to make sure you don't fully cook them) | Drain and run under cold water | Set aside

Peel and chop the onion and garlic | Rip the stem from the chili and chop, removing the seeds if you prefer a milder flavor | Trim the carrot and cut into matchsticks

Put the wok back over high heat and add the remaining 2 tablespoons of oil | Add the onion, garlic, and chili and cook, stirring regularly, for 1–2 minutes | Add the carrot and cook for another 1–2 minutes | Add the noodles, dressing, and a splash of water | Fry for a few minutes until the vegetables are tender

Return the tofu to the wok with the bean sprouts | Cut 1 lime in half and squeeze in the juice, catching any seeds in your other hand | Add the soy sauce | Stir-fry until the vegetables are slightly soft but still crunchy | Remove from the heat | Taste and add soy or chili sauce if needed

Slice the green part of the scallions into long, thin strips | Break up the peanuts | Cut the remaining limes into wedges

Divide the pad Thai among bowls with piles of sliced scallion, peanuts, lime wedges, and chili flakes | Serve with sweet chili sauce or sriracha on the side, if using

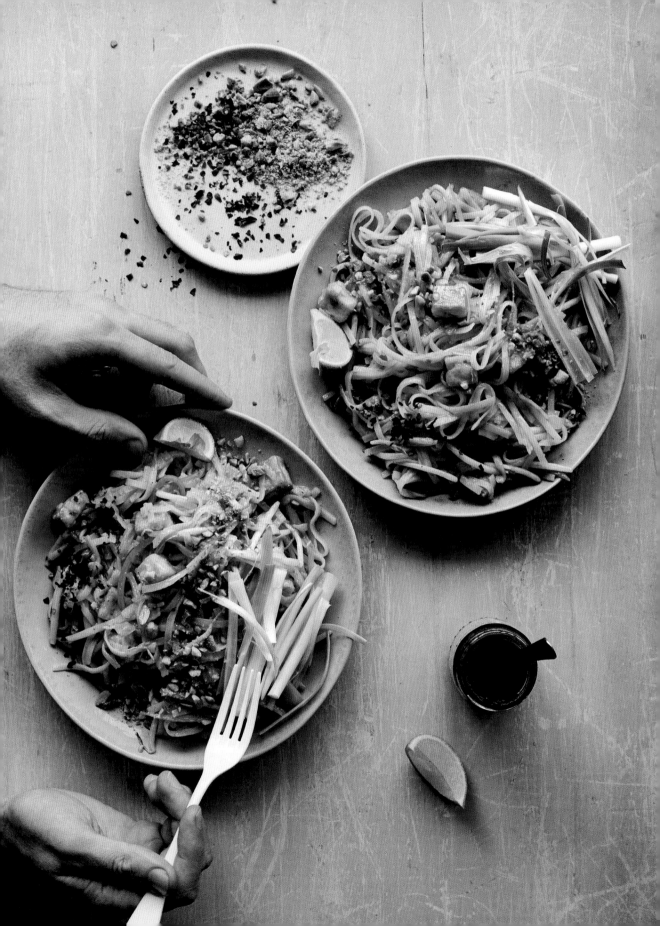

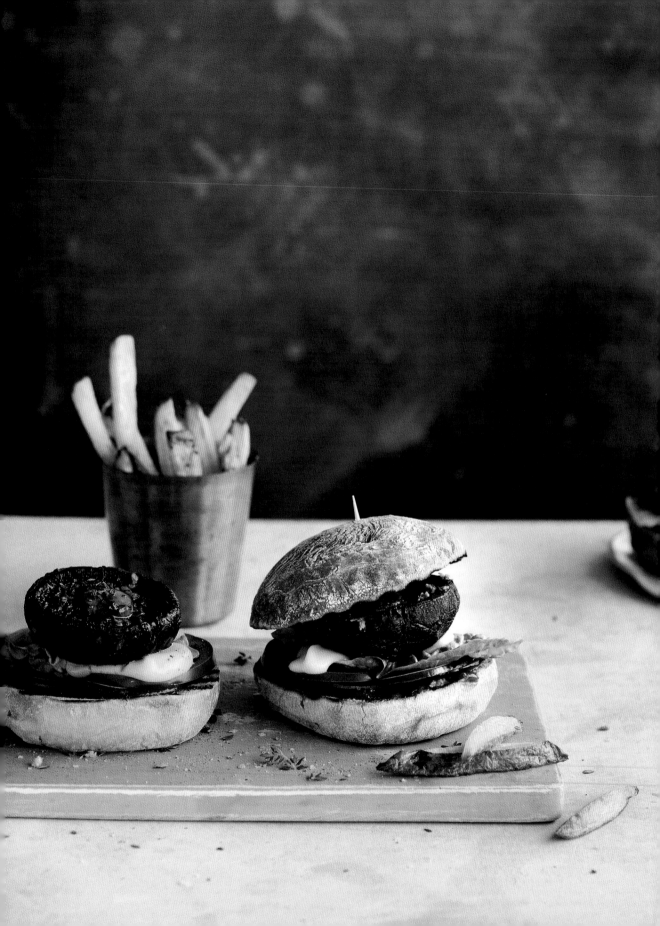

PORTOBELLO MUSHROOM BURGERS

The herbs are absolutely delicious in this dish and perfectly complement the earthy, rustic flavor of the portobello mushrooms. You could make these with pita bread if you want a healthier option, then fill the bread with as many veggies as you see fit.

SERVES 4

8 portobello mushrooms
4 garlic cloves
6 sprigs fresh thyme
3 sprigs fresh rosemary
4 tsp olive oil
4 tsp balsamic glaze
4 good-quality burger buns
1 beefsteak tomato
1 little gem lettuce
½ small red onion
¼ cup ketchup
¼ cup vegan mayonnaise
salt and black pepper

Preheat oven to 390°F or preheat a grill | Cut 8 squares of foil big enough to wrap your mushrooms | Baking sheet

Lay the mushrooms out on a clean surface with the stems pointing up | Peel and mince the garlic and spread it evenly over the mushrooms | Remove the leaves from the herbs by running your thumb and forefinger from the top to the base of the stems (the leaves should easily come away), then finely chop and sprinkle evenly over the mushrooms

Drizzle each mushroom with olive oil and balsamic glaze and lightly season with salt and pepper | Wrap each mushroom in a square of foil and place them on the baking sheet or on the hot grill | Put the baking sheet in the oven, if using, and cook for 20 minutes

Meanwhile, split the burger buns open | Slice the tomato, separate the lettuce leaves, and peel and thinly slice the onion | Drizzle some ketchup over the bottom of each bun and vegan mayo over the tops

Take the mushrooms out of the oven or off the grill | Carefully remove the foil (watch out for steam) and place 2 mushrooms on each bun bottom | Add the tomato slices, a couple of lettuce leaves, and a few slices of onion, put the tops on and enjoy

CRISPY CHILI TOFU

This is our take on one of our favorite Chinese take-out dishes. It's spicy, full of umami flavor, sticky, gooey, and incredibly moreish. Often when you buy this kind of dish it's filled with MSG, but ours is much healthier, with a base of orange juice and Thai sweet chili sauce adding the main sweet tang. Serve with Perfectly Boiled Rice (see page 207) or Special Fried Rice (see page 209).

SERVES 2–4

1 block (10 oz) firm tofu
1¼ cups cornstarch
vegetable oil, for frying
2 lemons
1 cup orange juice
6 tbsp Thai sweet chili sauce
1 tbsp sriracha or other chili-garlic sauce
3 tbsp soy sauce
1 scallion, to serve
1 tsp sesame seeds, to serve

Tofu press or 2 clean kitchen towels and a weight such as a heavy book | Large, deep frying pan over high heat | Large plate covered with paper towels

First, press the tofu using a tofu press or place it between two clean kitchen towels, lay it on a plate, and put a weight on top | Leave for at least 30 minutes to drain any liquid and firm up before you start cooking

Carefully slice the pressed tofu into sticks ⅓ inch wide and spread them out on a board | Sift cornstarch over the top, coating the pieces generously | Use tongs or two forks to turn the pieces and sift over more cornstarch until the tofu is covered on all sides | The thicker the better with the cornstarch as this coating gives the cooked tofu its crunchy texture

Pour enough oil into the pan to fully coat the bottom and heat until it makes the tip of a wooden spoon sizzle | Carefully place the tofu pieces in the pan, with a bit of space around each one (you may need to cook them in batches) | Cook for 5 minutes, turning the pieces every minute or so until they are starting to turn golden brown | Transfer to the plate lined with paper towels | Tip away the excess oil in the pan and reduce the heat to medium-high

Cut the lemons in half and squeeze the juice into the pan, catching any seeds in your other hand (be careful as the pan may spit) | Add the orange juice, sweet chili sauce, sriracha, and soy sauce and bring to a boil | Simmer for 5–7 minutes until the liquid has reduced to a syrupy consistency

Add the tofu strips back to the pan and stir until fully coated | Continue to cook, stirring regularly, for 5 minutes and then remove from the heat | Finely slice the scallion and sprinkle over the tofu along with the sesame seeds before serving

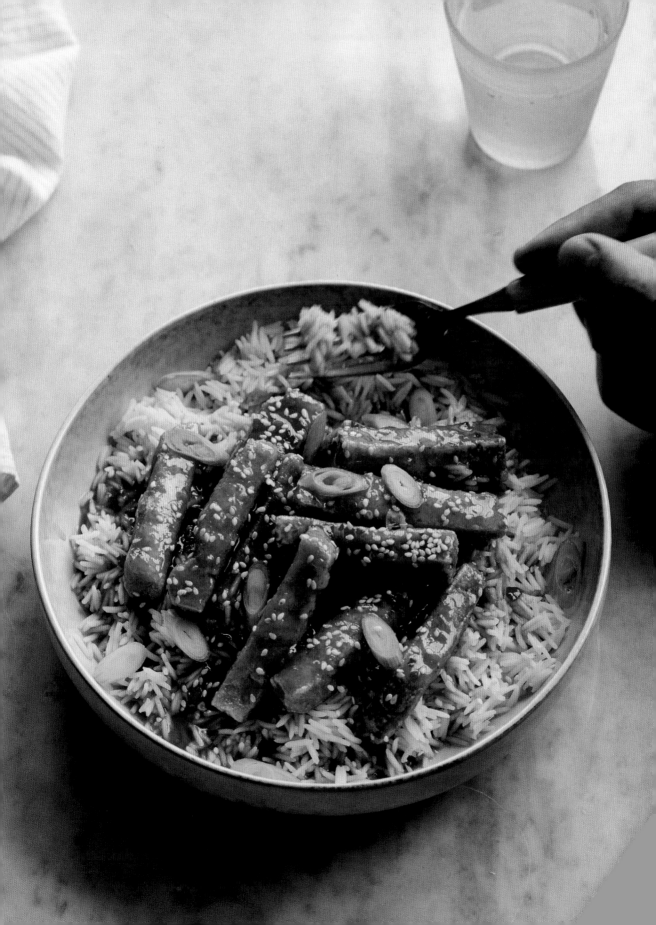

JACKFRUIT TACOS

Jackfruit is a fantastic and crowd-pleasing ingredient with a fibrous texture and flesh that soaks up flavor brilliantly, but it can be hard to find. Try your local Asian supermarket and be sure to choose green jackfruit in water. These tacos are perfect finger food, combining tasty jackfruit with a Mexican combo of zingy salsa and creamy guacamole.

SERVES 6

1 cup guacamole
  (store-bought or see page 194)
1 cup salsa (store-bought or see
  page 195)
1 can (14 oz) young green jackfruit
  in water
1 white onion
4 garlic cloves
1 tbsp vegetable oil
1 tbsp maple syrup
7 tbsp vegetable stock
½ tsp Tabasco sauce
4 limes
1½ tsp ground cumin
1½ tsp smoked paprika
½–1 tsp chili powder
½ tsp salt
handful fresh cilantro
12 crunchy taco shells

Deep frying pan with a lid over medium heat

If you're making your own guacamole and salsa, do this first following the instructions on pages 194 and 195

Tip the jackfruit into a sieve or colander to drain off the excess water and pat the pieces down with a clean kitchen towel to dry them off | Cut into ¼-inch strips and put to one side

Peel and slice the onion and garlic very thinly | Warm the vegetable oil in the frying pan | Add the onion and garlic to the pan and stir with a wooden spoon until soft and translucent | Add the jackfruit, maple syrup, vegetable stock, and Tabasco sauce | Cut 1 of the limes in half and squeeze in the juice of one half, catching any seeds in your other hand | Stir until the jackfruit is well covered

Put the lid on the pan, turn down the heat, and let it simmer for 7–10 minutes, stirring occasionally, until the liquid has been absorbed into the jackfruit | Take the lid off the pan and sprinkle in all the spices and the salt | Stir until the jackfruit pieces are well covered and taking on the color of the spices | Transfer the jackfruit pieces to a serving dish

Slice the remaining limes into wedges and remove the leaves from the cilantro by running your thumb and forefinger from the top to the base of the stems (the leaves should easily come away), saving the stems for another recipe | Serve the taco shells, jackfruit, guacamole, salsa, lime wedges, and cilantro leaves on individual plates and let everyone build their own tacos

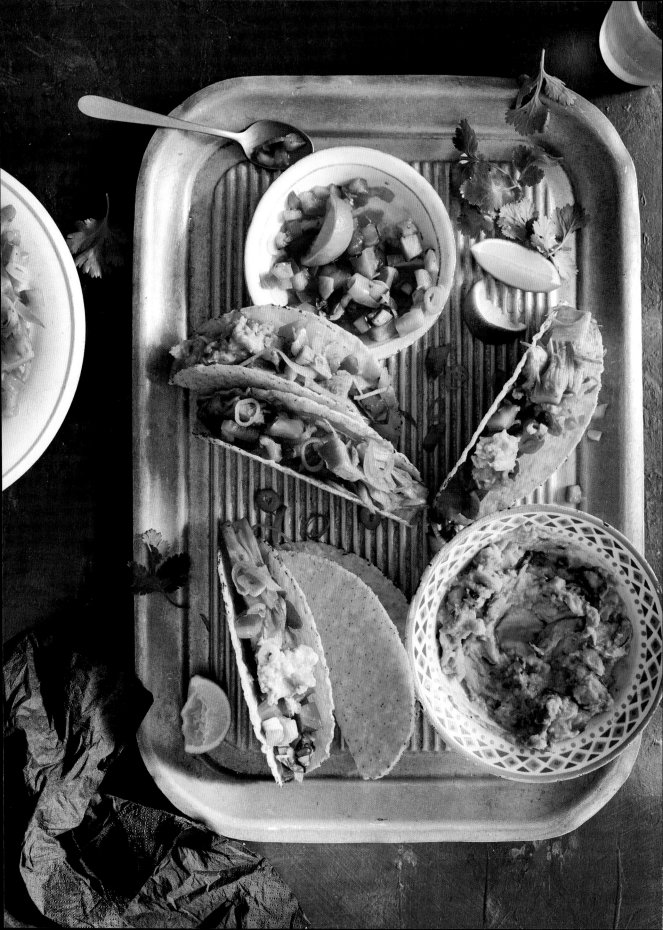

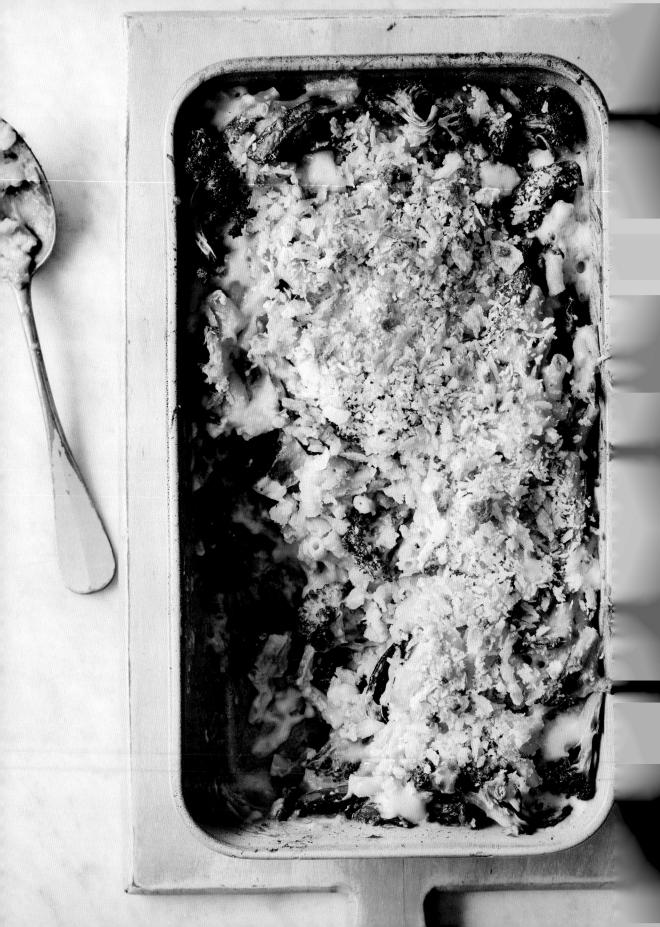

CREAMY MAC & GREENS

This is our take on one of the world's most popular tasty treats, a crowd-pleasing classic. A béchamel sauce makes it creamy and delicious and then we add a rich, salty flavor with roasted mushrooms. This dish is moreish and indulgent, and healthy(ish), and makes a great main course or side for a BBQ.

SERVES 6

1 head of broccoli
1 red onion
2 tbsp olive oil
8 portobello mushrooms (about 12 oz)
12 oz macaroni
3 cups unsweetened plant-based milk
5 tbsp dairy-free butter or spread
7 tbsp all-purpose flour
2 tsp onion powder
1½ tsp garlic powder
2 tsp prepared English mustard
¼ cup nutritional yeast
1½ oz dairy-free cheese, grated
1¼ tsp salt, plus a little extra
¾ tsp black pepper, plus a little extra
scant ½ cup panko breadcrumbs
salad leaves, to serve, optional

FOR THE MARINADE
5 tbsp soy sauce
1 tbsp plus 1 tsp maple syrup
1 tbsp plus 1 tsp apple cider vinegar
1 tbsp plus 1 tsp olive oil

Preheat oven to 350°F | Line 2 baking sheets | Large saucepan of salted water over high heat | Medium saucepan over medium heat | 9 x 13-inch baking dish

Cut the broccoli into roughly 1-inch florets and cubes (trim the stems and use the soft parts) | Peel and roughly chop the onion into ⅓-inch chunks | Lay both the onion and broccoli on one of the lined baking sheets, drizzle with the 2 tablespoons of olive oil, and lightly season with salt and pepper | Put the sheet on the top shelf of the preheated oven

Cut the mushrooms into ⅓-inch chunks | Put the ingredients for the marinade into a bowl and combine with a fork | Add the mushroom pieces to the marinade and stir to coat | Spread the mushrooms over the second lined baking sheet and put this in the oven on the shelf below the broccoli and onions | Set the timer for 15 minutes, by which time all the veggies should be golden brown | Remove both baking sheets and increase the oven temperature to 425°F

While the vegetables are roasting, add the macaroni to the pan of boiling salted water and cook until al dente, according to the package directions | Drain and tip into the baking dish

Meanwhile, warm the plant-based milk in the microwave | Put the dairy-free butter in the medium saucepan and stir with a wooden spoon until it melts | Turn the heat right down and gradually add the flour to the pan, stirring vigorously until you have a doughy paste | Gradually pour in the warm plant-based milk, stirring all the time until you have a thick, creamy sauce | Add the onion powder, garlic powder, mustard powder, nutritional yeast, dairy-free cheese, 1¼ teaspoons salt, and ¾ teaspoon pepper and stir into the sauce | Keep stirring until the sauce thickens to the consistency of custard

Add the cooked vegetables and sauce to the pasta and mix together so that everything is well covered | Sprinkle the breadcrumbs over the top, season with salt and pepper, and put the dish in the oven for 5 minutes to warm through and crisp up the breadcrumbs | Remove from the oven and serve with a small side salad, if you like

STIR-FRY NOODLES

Stir-fries are great go-to dishes for any night of the week. Once you've mastered a few different recipes you can knock out a tasty, healthy, satisfying meal in minutes, using whatever you've got left in the fridge. Become a stir-fry ninja and a world of culinary deliciousness awaits you.

1. **Drop 2 tablespoons oil into a hot wok**
   Canola oil
   Coconut oil
   Olive oil
   Toasted sesame oil
   Vegetable oil

2. **Trim and finely chop your aromatics and add them to the pan**
   Garlic
   Ginger
   Red chili
   Shallots
   Scallions

3. **Trim and finely slice the vegetables and add them to the pan (¾ lb total veggies will serve 4 people)**
   Asparagus
   Baby corn
   Bean sprouts
   Bell peppers
   Bok choy
   Broccoli
   Celery
   Mushrooms
   Onion
   Snow peas
   Spinach
   Sugar snap peas
   Zucchini

4. **Prepare your noodles following the package directions (they might need cooking before they go into the wok) and fold them into the vegetables (12 oz noodles will serve 4 people)**
   Glass noodles
   Rice noodles
   Rice vermicelli
   Soba noodles
   Udon noodles
   Whole wheat noodles

5. **Drizzle your sauce over the vegetables and stir everything together**
   Basic Stir-fry (see opposite)
   Orange & Ginger (see opposite)
   Black Pepper (see opposite)
   Sweet & Sour (see opposite)
   Hoisin
   Soy
   Teriyaki

6. **Season your stir-fry and transfer to plates**
   Lemon
   Lime
   Salt

7. **Finish off your stir-fry with the garnish of your choice**
   Cashews
   Cilantro leaves
   Hot sauce
   Peanuts
   Scallions, chopped
   Sesame seeds

SAUCE RECIPES

It's crucial to get an awesome sauce, but it doesn't need to be complicated; whatever you have in your kitchen will serve just fine, or you can knock together one of our sauces below for an extra kick of deliciousness!

BASIC STIR-FRY

SERVES 4

3 garlic cloves
1 tbsp brown sugar
2 tsp cornstarch
7 tbsp vegetable stock
3 tbsp soy sauce
1 tbsp rice vinegar

Peel and finely chop the garlic | Put all the ingredients for your sauce into a measuring cup and mix together with a fork

SWEET & SOUR

SERVES 4

1 tbsp brown sugar
2 tsp cornstarch
½ cup vegetable stock
2 tbsp ketchup
1 tbsp soy sauce
1 tbsp rice vinegar

Put all the ingredients for your sauce into a measuring cup and mix together with a fork

ORANGE & GINGER

SERVES 4

1¼-inch piece fresh ginger
2 tsp cornstarch
3 tbsp soy sauce
1 tbsp rice wine vinegar
juice of 1 large orange

Peel the ginger by scraping off the skin with a spoon and finely chop | Put all the ingredients for your sauce into a measuring cup and mix together with a fork

BLACK PEPPER

SERVES 4

7 tbsp vegetable stock
1 tbsp cornstarch
2 tbsp water
1 tsp brown sugar
1 tsp black pepper
3 tbsp soy sauce
2 tsp rice vinegar

Put all the ingredients for your sauce into a measuring cup and mix together with a fork

02

BIG
EATS

Cook a proper meal
Spend that extra time on food
To please and delight

MUSHROOM & GUINNESS PIE

Oh my goodness, this take on a pub classic is so so good. It's a hug in a dish! The mushroom is rich and meaty and the Guinness adds a dark umami flavor. It's one for those winter nights after a long day in the cold (or at work!). Serve with Minted Mushy Peas (see page 136).

SERVES 4–6

1½ lb cremini mushrooms

3 tbsp olive oil

4 onions

6 garlic cloves

3 sprigs fresh rosemary, plus extra to decorate

3 sprigs fresh thyme

1 tbsp light brown sugar

1¼ cups Guinness or other stout or brown ale

2½ tbsp all-purpose flour, plus extra for dusting

1–2 tbsp Dijon mustard

5 tsp dark soy sauce

1 lb ready-made dairy-free puff pastry

2 tbsp dairy-free margarine

salt and black pepper

Preheat oven to 350°F | Line a rimmed baking sheet | Large frying pan over medium heat | 8 to 8½-inch deep-dish pie plate | Rolling pin (or use a clean, dry wine bottle) | Pastry brush

Quarter the mushrooms and spread them over the lined baking sheet | Drizzle with 1 tablespoon of the oil, season lightly, and roast in the preheated oven for 15 minutes | When they're ready, remove and set aside, reserving any juices

Meanwhile, add the remaining 2 tablespoons of oil to the frying pan | Peel and slice the onions | Peel and finely chop the garlic | Add to the pan and cook for 10 minutes, stirring occasionally, until softened | Reduce the temperature to medium-low

Remove the leaves from the rosemary and thyme by running your thumb and forefinger from the top to the base of the stems (the leaves should easily come away) and finely chop, discarding the stems | Add to the pan along with the sugar and cook for 10 more minutes, until the onions are golden

Pour the ale into the pan, bring to a simmer, and cook for 10 more minutes so the liquid reduces | Reduce the heat to low and add the mushrooms and any juices in the baking sheet | Add the flour, mustard, and soy sauce and simmer gently for 15–20 minutes, stirring regularly | Taste and adjust the seasoning, adding more salt, pepper, mustard, or soy sauce if you like | Leave to cool slightly, then spoon the mushroom mixture into the pie plate

Lightly dust a work surface with flour and roll out the pastry until it is large enough to cover the top of the pie plate | Brush the rim of the dish with water and lay the pastry over the top | Cut off the excess pastry and crimp the edges of the pastry either by pinching it between your finger and thumb all the way round, or by pressing it against the dish with the back of a fork

Melt the dairy-free margarine in the microwave and brush it all over the pastry | Use a small sharp knife to cut a little cross in the center of the pastry so that steam can escape | Top with a few rosemary sprigs to make it look fancy | Bake in the preheated oven for 30–35 minutes, until the pastry is golden brown, remove, and serve hot

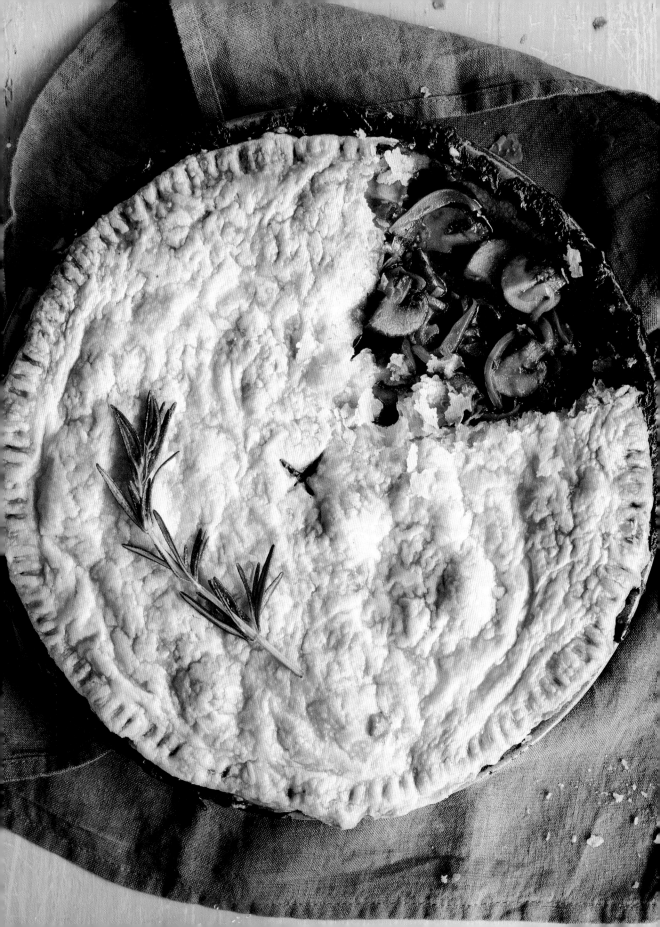

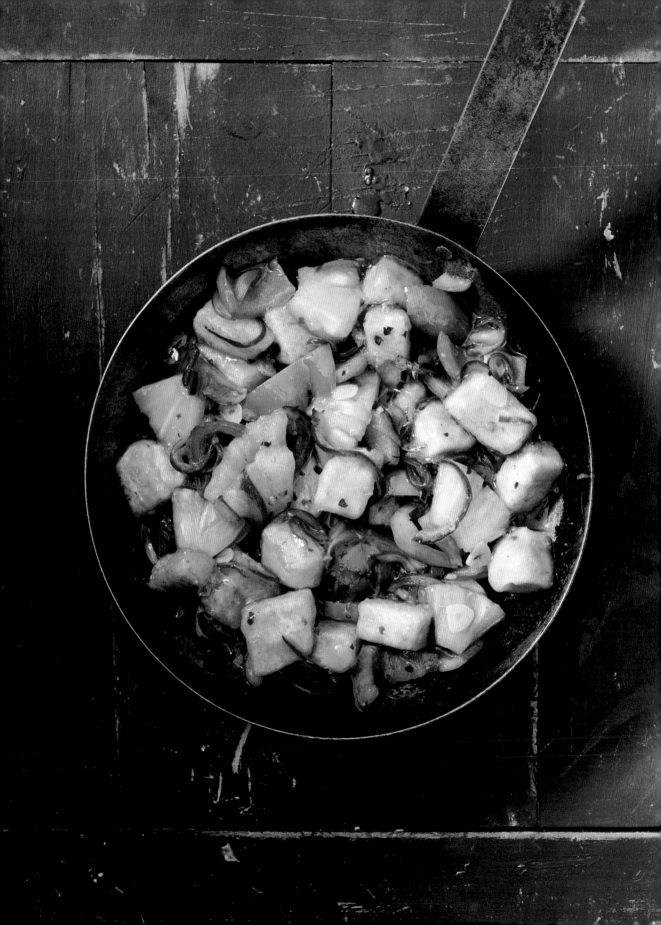

SWEET & SOUR CRISPY TOFU

Sweet and sour needs no introduction! This dish is an indulgent worldwide classic made with smooth, soft tofu. It's made even more delicious by the addition of pineapple, and the way the crispy fried tofu contrasts with the sweet syrupy sauce. Mix this with any other Asian dish and boiled rice and you have a winner on your hands.

SERVES 2–4

block (10 oz) firm tofu
2½-inch piece fresh ginger
1 red onion
1 garlic clove
1 green bell pepper
generous ¾ cup pineapple juice
¼ cup rice vinegar
¼ cup ketchup
6 tbsp light brown sugar
1 tsp garlic powder
1 tsp onion powder, optional
¼ cup cornstarch
2 tbsp vegetable oil
2 tbsp toasted sesame oil
½ tsp chili flakes
½ tsp salt
⅔ cup canned pineapple chunks

Small saucepan over medium-low heat | Tofu press or 2 clean kitchen towels and a weight such as a heavy book | 2 large frying pans over medium-high heat | Fine grater

Press the tofu using a tofu press, or place it between two clean kitchen towels, lay it on a plate, and put a weight on top | Leave for at least 30 minutes to drain any liquid and firm up before you start cooking

Peel the ginger by scraping off the skin with a spoon and then grate it | Peel and finely slice the red onion and the garlic | Cut the bell pepper in half and cut out the stem and seeds | Chop the pepper into ¾-inch chunks

Put the pineapple juice, rice vinegar, ketchup, and brown sugar in the small saucepan and stir to dissolve the sugar | Increase the heat to medium-high and let it bubble away for about 7 minutes until you have a syrupy sauce | Take the saucepan off the heat and set aside

Put the garlic powder and the onion powder, if using, into a large bowl with the cornstarch and mix together | Carefully cut the drained tofu into ⅓-inch chunks and add them to the bowl | Toss them gently in the cornstarch mixture until they're well covered

Heat the vegetable oil in one of the large frying pans | Add the tofu chunks and fry until they have started to brown and formed a crispy coating, about 7–10 minutes (be delicate as you stir the cubes, you want to keep them intact) | Take the pan off the heat and set aside

Meanwhile, heat the sesame oil in the second frying pan | Add the onion slices and stir until translucent, about 5 minutes | Add the bell pepper, chili flakes, salt, garlic, and ginger and continue to cook for another 3–5 minutes, stirring all the time | Drain the pineapple and add to the pan, continuing to stir until the pineapple is warm | Tip the tofu into the pan and heat | Pour in the sweet and sour sauce and fold it around the vegetables so that everything is well covered and warmed through, another 1–2 minutes

IRRESISTIBLE RISOTTO

This risotto is bursting with color, flavor, and healthy goodness. We're big fans of getting as much green into our bodies as possible to give us the vital nutrients we need. This dish is testament to that, but it's also delicious. Cook slowly, add the stock bit by bit, and you'll have a dish guaranteed to please!

SERVES 4

2 oz macadamia nuts
1 medium red onion
2 large garlic cloves
3 tbsp mixed fresh herbs, such as sage, parsley, and mint
2½ oz green beans
2 oz asparagus
2 oz kale
½ lemon
3¾ cups vegetable stock
2 tbsp olive oil
1 cup + 2 tbsp risotto rice, such as Arborio or Carnaroli
½ cup dry white wine
generous ½ cup green peas
3 tbsp nutritional yeast
1½ tbsp dairy-free butter or spread
salt and black pepper

Preheat oven to 325°F | Small baking sheet | Medium saucepan over low heat | Medium saucepan over medium heat

Spread the macadamia nuts over the small baking sheet, put the pan in the oven, and toast for 5–8 minutes, until golden | Leave to cool slightly, then roughly chop

Meanwhile, peel and finely chop the red onion and garlic | Chop the herbs | Slice the green beans into ¾-inch pieces | Snap the tough ends off the asparagus and cut the stalks into ⅓-inch pieces | Remove the tough stems from the kale and roughly chop | Finely grate the zest of the lemon

Pour the stock into the medium saucepan over low heat and keep warm

Add the olive oil to the other pan | Add the chopped onions and cook until they begin to soften, about 10–15 minutes | Add the garlic and stir for another minute | Pour in the rice and toast for a minute longer

Turn up the heat slightly and pour in the white wine | Simmer until the liquid has almost completely evaporated, stirring frequently | Add the green beans and asparagus to the pan and give everything a stir

Now start adding a ladleful of stock at a time, stirring continuously and waiting for the stock to be absorbed before adding the next ladleful | After 8 minutes, add the peas and kale to the pan and continue to cook for 6–8 minutes longer, until the rice is just cooked and the vegetables are tender (you might have a little stock left over)

Remove the pan from the heat, stir in the chopped herbs, nutritional yeast, lemon zest, macadamia nuts, and dairy-free butter | Season to taste with salt and pepper and serve immediately

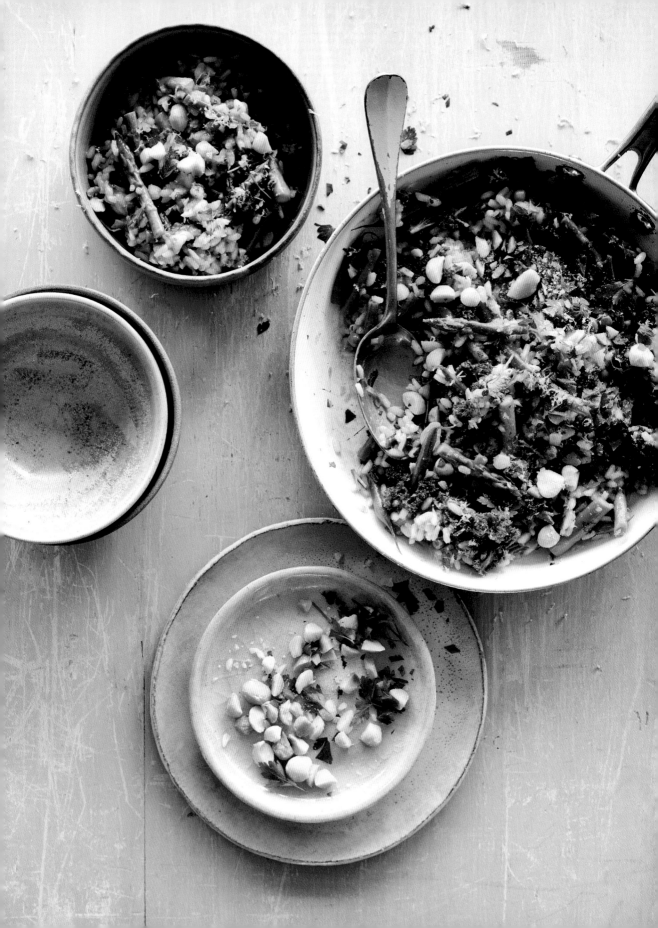

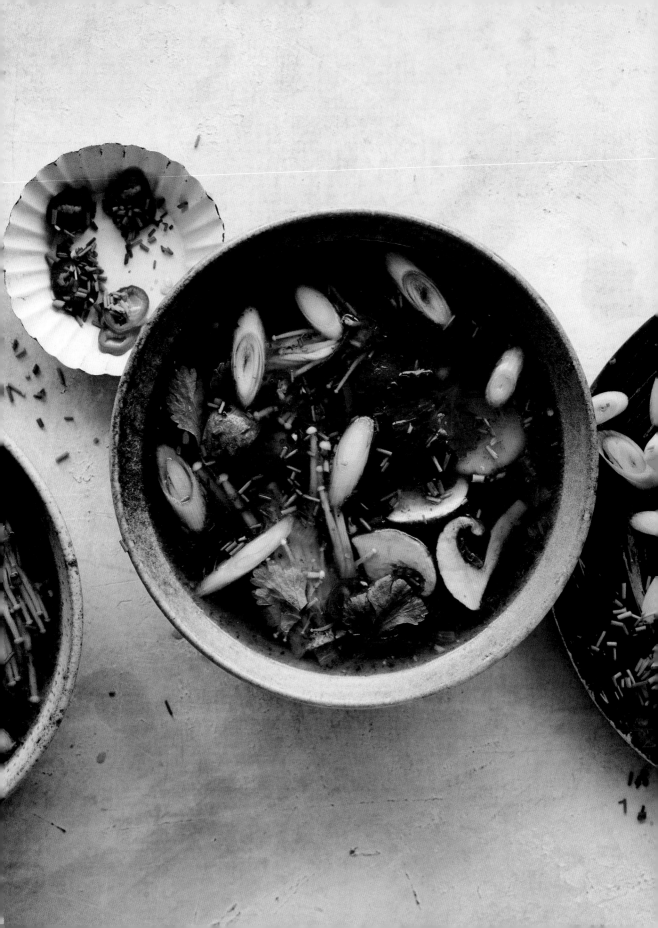

TOM YUM SOUP

This was Henry's dish of choice as he traveled around Thailand. The healthy, spicy Thai classic just feels like holiday. As a soup it's surprisingly filling, and it's best eaten when it's so hot and spicy it's hard to continue and you break into sweats! Slurping is good here. Let this gorgeously hot, spicy soup warm you to your core!

SERVES 4

¼ cup olive oil
1 small onion
4 garlic cloves
2 fresh red chilies
1-inch piece fresh ginger
6 cups vegetable stock
1 tsp tomato paste
2 lemongrass stalks
6 kaffir lime leaves
2 limes
9 oz cremini mushrooms
3½ oz enoki mushrooms (2 bunches)
7 oz cherry tomatoes
1 can (8 oz) water chestnuts, optional
4 scallions, to serve
small handful fresh chives, to serve
small handful fresh cilantro, to serve

FOR THE TOM YUM PASTE
2 tbsp vegetable oil
¼ cup Thai Red Curry Paste (see page 78)
3 tbsp palm sugar
1 tsp salt

Wok over medium heat

First make the tom yum paste | Add the vegetable oil to the wok | When it's hot add the red curry paste, palm sugar, and salt and fry for 3 minutes, until the paste goes a darker red color | Remove from the heat and scrape into a bowl | Give the wok a quick rinse and put back on the heat

Add the olive oil to the clean wok | Peel and roughly chop the onion | Peel the garlic | Rip the stems from the chilies and finely slice one, removing the seeds if you prefer a milder flavor | Peel the ginger by scraping off the skin with a spoon and finely chop | Crush the garlic into the wok, add in the onion, chili, and ginger, and cook for 4 minutes to allow the flavors to infuse

Pour 2 cups of the stock into the wok and bring to a boil | Add the tom yum paste and mix well | Add the remaining stock and the tomato paste | Bash the bases of the lemongrass stalks and add them to the pan | Slice the lime leaves and throw them in | Simmer for 20 minutes

Cut the limes in half and squeeze in the juice, catching any seeds in your other hand | Halve the cremini mushrooms and add them to the pan with the enoki mushrooms and the tomatoes | Slice the water chestnuts, if using, and add them to the pan | Finely slice the remaining chili into long diagonal slices, removing the seeds if you prefer a milder flavor, and add to the pan | Simmer for 5 minutes longer

Divide the soup among bowls | Trim and slice the scallions and chop the chives | Sprinkle over the soup along with the cilantro leaves and serve

PASTA CAPONATA

This hearty dish features a rich Sicilian caponata sauce, complete with pine nuts and raisins, which has great depth of flavor, but with an added celery crunch and kick of chili. Feel free to use more or less garlic (we like lots of garlic!) and then serve with bread to soak up all the juices.

SERVES 4–6

2 eggplants (about 1 lb)
10 oz cherry tomatoes
3 tbsp olive oil
1½ tsp chili flakes
1 red onion
3 garlic cloves
1 celery stalk
2 tbsp tomato paste
1 can (14.5 oz) chopped tomatoes
1 tsp dried oregano
2 sprigs fresh thyme
3 tbsp small capers
¼ cup raisins
2 oz pitted Kalamata olives
1 lb penne pasta
½ oz dark chocolate
20 sprigs fresh parsley
1 tbsp balsamic vinegar
1½ oz pine nuts
salt and black pepper

Preheat oven to 350°F | Line a baking sheet | Large frying pan with lid over medium heat | Large saucepan | Small frying pan

Trim the eggplants and chop the flesh into ¾-inch cubes | Lay on the lined baking sheet along with the cherry tomatoes and drizzle over 1 tablespoon of the olive oil | Sprinkle with a good layer of salt, pepper, and the chili flakes, put the pan in the preheated oven, and bake for 30 minutes

Meanwhile, pour the remaining 2 tablespoons of oil into the large frying pan | Peel and finely chop the onion and garlic and add to the pan | Trim the leaves and root from the celery, then finely chop and add to the pan | Cook the onions, garlic, and celery for 10–15 minutes, stirring regularly, until they are soft and translucent

Add the tomato paste to the pan and stir | Add the chopped tomatoes, oregano, thyme, capers, raisins, and olives, plus a little salt and pepper to taste, then reduce the heat to a gentle simmer and let everything cook for 5 minutes | Remove the roasted eggplants and tomatoes from the oven and add them to the pan, giving everything a stir | Put the lid on and simmer for 12–15 minutes, stirring every 5 minutes to stop it burning

Bring a large saucepan of water to a boil and add a pinch of salt | Add the pasta and cook until al dente, according to the package directions | Drain the pasta and tip the cooked pasta back into the pasta pan

Meanwhile, chop or grate the dark chocolate and sprinkle it into the caponata sauce | Strip the parsley leaves from the stems (save the stems for another recipe), then chop the leaves and add three-quarters to the pan along with the balsamic vinegar | Simmer uncovered for 3–5 minutes longer | Taste and season if necessary | Pour the sauce over the pasta and fold it in, making sure everything is well covered

Put the small frying pan over medium-high heat and toast the pine nuts in the dry pan until golden | Sprinkle over the pasta along with the remaining parsley leaves before serving

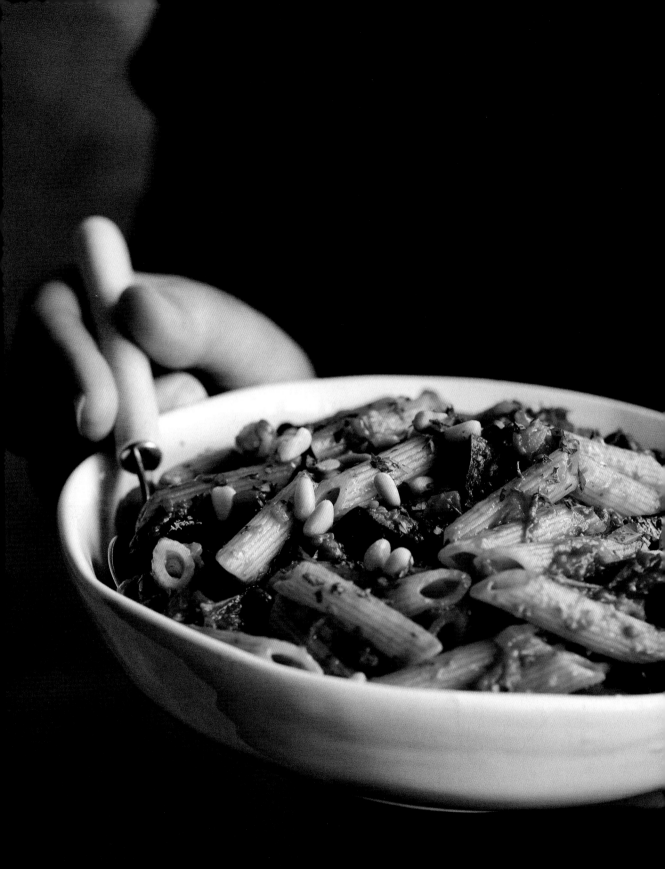

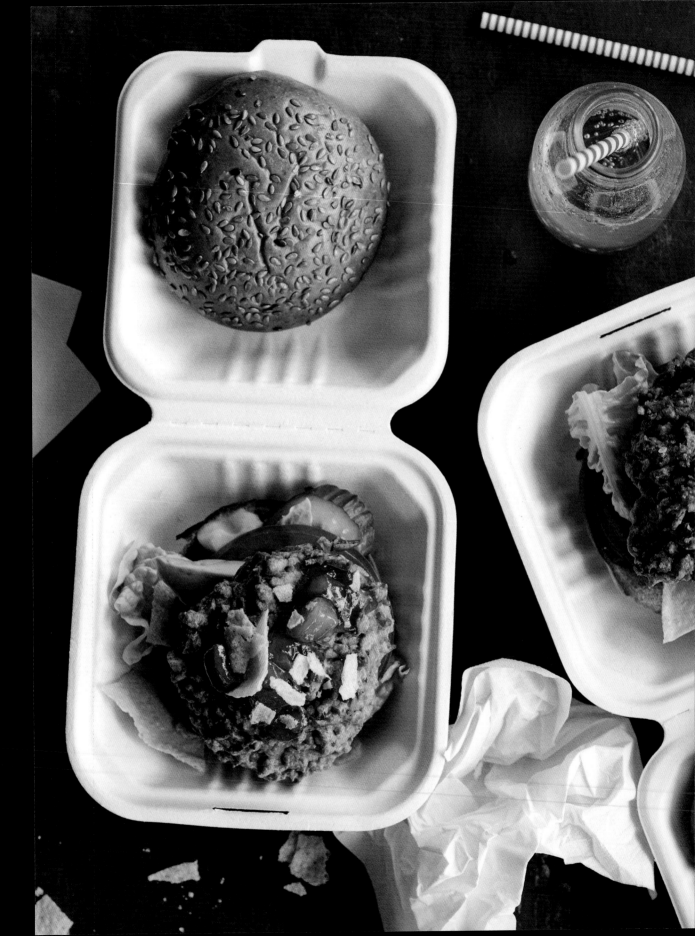

BIG BHAJI BURGER

This juxtaposition of Indian cuisine with the classic American burger works incredibly well. It's a fantastic fusion of flavors that are really big and satisfying, and you can play with really interesting toppings. These are great with Jane's Mint Raita (see page 204), or make smaller bhaji bites and serve them with curry.

MAKES 6

2–4 cups vegetable oil, for
    deep-frying
2 red onions
2½-inch piece fresh ginger
1 fresh red chili
generous 1 cup fresh cilantro leaves
1½ tsp coriander seeds
1½ tsp cumin seeds
2½ cups chickpea flour
1½ tsp garam masala
generous ¾ cup water
4 good-quality burger buns
3 tbsp vegan mayonnaise, to serve
¼ small cucumber, to serve
1 large tomato, to serve
1 avocado, to serve
1 little gem lettuce, to serve
2 tbsp mango chutney, to serve
1 pappadum, to serve
salt

Large saucepan over high heat | Cooking thermometer, optional | Pestle and mortar | Line a dinner plate with paper towels

Pour the vegetable oil into the large saucepan so that it comes no more than two-thirds up the side of the pan | Heat the oil to 350°F, or until a wooden spoon dipped into the oil sizzles around the edges

Meanwhile, peel and very finely slice the onions and put them into a big bowl | Peel the ginger by scraping off the skin with a spoon and finely chop | Rip the stem from the chili, cut it in half lengthwise, and remove the seeds if you prefer a milder flavor, then finely chop and add to the pan | Roughly chop the cilantro leaves | Add the ginger, chili, and cilantro to the bowl | Crush the coriander seeds and cumin seeds with a pestle and mortar or the end of a rolling pin and add them to the bowl | Add the chickpea flour, garam masala, water, and a generous pinch of salt and mix until everything is well combined and covered with a wet sticky batter

Divide the mixture into 6 and use your hands to mold it into patties around 3½ inches wide and no more than ⅓ inch thick | Use a metal spoon to carefully lower 2 of the patties into the hot oil and cook them for about 5 minutes, flipping them over halfway | Remove the patties when they are golden and crisp and transfer to the plate lined with paper towels to drain any excess oil | Repeat with the remaining patties

While the bhajis are frying, split the burger buns open and spread the bottom halves with vegan mayonnaise | Thinly slice the cucumber and tomato | Halve and carefully pit the avocado by tapping the pit firmly with the heel of a knife so that it lodges in the pit, then twist and remove the pit | Run a spoon around the inside of the avocado skin to scoop out the flesh, then slice finely

To serve the bhaji burgers, lay a few lettuce leaves on the bottom of the burger buns and place the burgers on top | Spread a little mango chutney on top of each, followed by slices of tomato, avocado, and cucumber | Break up the pappadum and sprinkle it over the top before closing the buns

CREAMY SEASIDE PIE

Nothing says "taste of the British seaside" more than a fish pie, so we've replicated that flavor with a clever combination of mushrooms, capers, and lemon. Topped with crispy but fluffy potato, this hearty, healthy dish is guaranteed to impress your guests and warm your cockles. The different mushroom shapes give a wonderfully varied texture to this dish, just like a fish pie.

SERVES 6

1 large white onion

4 garlic cloves

1 lb 5 oz mixed mushrooms (this works best with Japanese mushrooms like shiitake, oyster mushrooms, buna shimeji, shiro shimeji, eryngii or king oysters, enoki, golden enoki, maitake, or a mixture)

3 tbsp olive oil

2 sheets nori

7 tbsp white wine

1 tbsp salt, plus a little extra

3 tbsp unsweetened plant-based milk

1 tbsp whole-grain mustard

2 tbsp nutritional yeast

2 tbsp capers

1 tbsp caper brine

1 lemon

¾ cup soy cream

1½ cups frozen green peas

1 oz parsley leaves

black pepper

FOR THE POTATO TOPPING

3 lb russet or other fluffy potatoes

3 tbsp dairy-free butter or spread, plus a little extra

½ cup soy cream

3 tbsp unsweetened plant-based milk

1 tsp whole-grain mustard

1 tbsp nutritional yeast

salt and black pepper

Preheat oven to 350°F | Large, deep frying pan over medium heat | Large saucepan with lid | 9 x 13-inch baking dish

To make the topping, peel the potatoes and cut into large chunks | Put them in the large saucepan and add enough cold water to cover them | Add a big pinch of salt | Turn the heat to high and bring the water to a boil, then cover the pan partially with a lid and simmer for 15–20 minutes, until the potatoes are tender when pierced with a knife | Drain in a colander, then tip the potatoes back into the pan and set aside

Meanwhile, peel and finely chop the onion and the garlic and roughly chop the mushrooms | Warm the oil in the large frying pan | Add the chopped onions to the pan and cook for 10 minutes, until soft (cook them slowly to make sure they don't burn and to draw out the flavor)

Use scissors to cut the nori into ⅓-inch pieces and sprinkle them into the pan | Increase the heat to medium-high and add the chopped garlic and mushrooms | Cook for about 10 minutes, until soft, slightly golden, and significantly reduced in size (the pan will be very full to start) | Pour in the white wine and cook until reduced by half, another 2–3 minutes

Reduce the heat to medium and add 1 tablespoon of salt, the plant-based milk, mustard, and the nutritional yeast | Add the capers and the tablespoon of brine from the jar | Cut the lemon in half and squeeze in the juice, catching any seeds with your other hand | Stir everything around and continue to cook until the mushrooms have soaked up around half the liquid, about 10 minutes | Pour the soy cream into the pan and stir everything together so that the sauce has a nice creamy texture

Add the peas to the pan, folding them in so that they're well mixed | Take the pan off the heat | Roughly chop the parsley and stir it into the mixture | Pour the mushroom filling into the baking dish

Return to the potatoes | Add the dairy-free butter, soy cream, plant-based milk, mustard, and nutritional yeast to the potatoes and mash together until thick and creamy | Taste and season with salt and pepper

Spoon the mashed potato on top of the mushroom filling and carefully smooth it out to the edges of the dish | Use a fork to scrape lines across the top | Flake over bits of dairy-free butter, if you like, to help the potato crisp up | Put in the oven and bake for 20 minutes, then put under the broiler for 2–3 minutes so it has a crispy crust with golden brown peaks

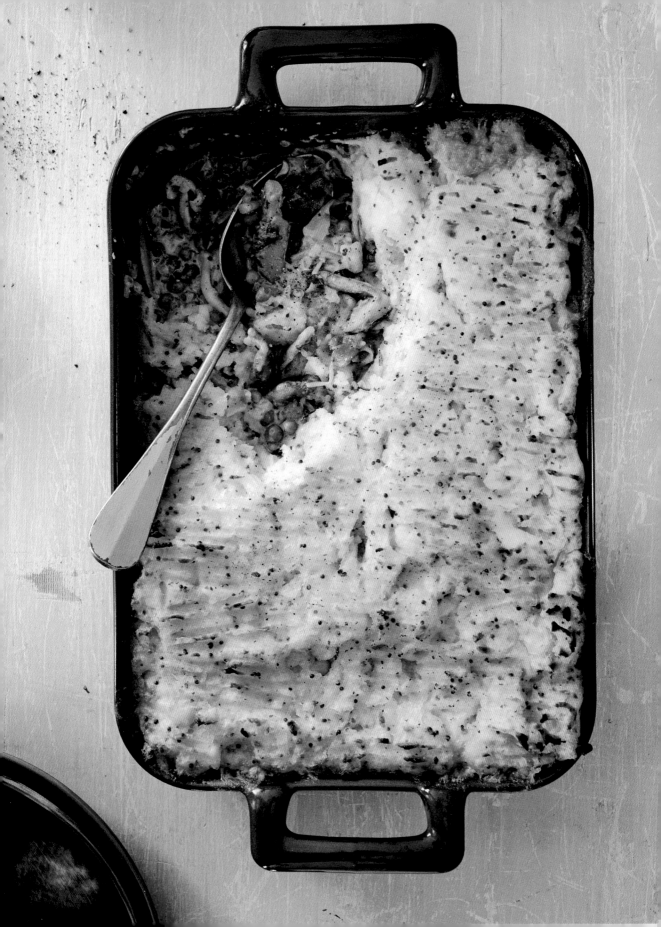

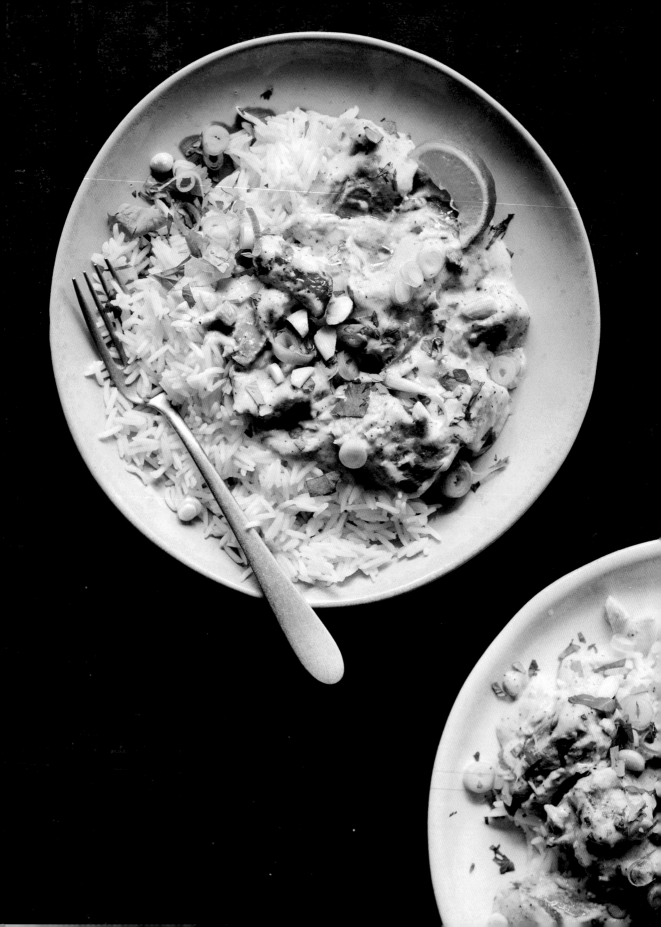

CREAMY KORMA

Korma is often thought of as an accessible beginner's curry. But, let's be honest, that's because it's downright delicious. We love a creamy korma. It's a dish that's close to our hearts. This one is healthy, tasty, and full of hearty flavor. Trust us, you're going to love it. Feel free to use any combination of roast vegetables you like. Serve with rice (see page 207) or Naan (see page 203).

SERVES 4–6

1 large sweet potato (about 14 oz)
½ butternut squash (about 1 lb)
2 carrots (about 5 oz)
3 tbsp vegetable oil
2 large white onions
7 green cardamom pods
1½ tsp poppy seeds
2 whole cloves
1 bay leaf
1¾ oz cashews
2½ oz blanched almonds
¾-inch piece fresh ginger
2 fresh green chilies
3 garlic cloves
½ tsp ground nutmeg
½ tsp ground turmeric
1 can (14 oz) coconut milk
2 limes
cooked rice, to serve, optional
small bunch of fresh cilantro, to serve
2 scallions, to serve
salt

Preheat oven to 350°F | Line a baking sheet | Blender | Large frying pan

Peel the sweet potato, squash and carrots | Cut into ¾-inch chunks and arrange on the lined baking sheet | Drizzle with 1 tablespoon of the oil and season lightly with salt | Put the pan in the oven and roast for 30 minutes, turning the pan in the oven after 20 minutes if necessary | Remove when softened and a little brown | Peel and finely slice the onions

Bash the cardamom pods with the end of a knife and tear them open | Tip the seeds into the large frying pan | Add the poppy seeds and cloves and set over medium-high heat | Toast for 2 minutes

Reduce the heat to medium-low | Add the remaining 2 tablespoons of oil | Add the onions, bay leaf, cashews, and three-quarters of the blanched almonds | Stir and cook for 12 minutes, until the onions are soft and the nuts slightly golden, stirring regularly

Peel the ginger by scraping off the skin with a spoon, then roughly chop | Rip the stems from the chilies, cut them in half lengthwise, and remove the seeds if you prefer a milder sauce, then finely chop | Peel and crush the garlic into the pan | Add the ginger, chili, ground nutmeg, and turmeric to the pan | Cook for another 2 minutes

Take off the heat and cool for 5 minutes | Remove the bay leaf | Transfer to the blender with half the coconut milk and whizz to a smooth paste, about 60 seconds | Pour back into the pan and set over medium heat

Add the roasted vegetables to the pan | Pour in the rest of the coconut milk and stir gently until well mixed | Reduce the heat and simmer for about 5 minutes | Add a splash of water if the sauce is too thick

Cut the limes in half and squeeze the juice over the curry, catching any seeds in your other hand | Season to taste with salt

Divide among 4–6 plates and serve with rice, if using | Chop the stems from the cilantro and save for another recipe, then chop the leaves and the rest of the blanched almonds and slice the scallions | Scatter a little over each portion

PASTABALL MARINARA

This inside-out pasta dish is insanely delicious! We were coming up with revolutionary burger recipes and, like Einstein creating relativity, realized we could make meatballs out of pasta. The tomato sauce is one of the lushest, thickest pasta sauces we have ever created—it's truly scrumptious. If you prefer less sugar, substitute vegan pesto for the BBQ sauce.

SERVES 4

9 oz whole-wheat pasta shapes, such as penne
1 can (15 oz) black beans
1¾ oz sun-dried tomatoes in oil
1 tbsp chili powder
3 tbsp BBQ sauce
olive oil
1 large onion
2 garlic cloves
a few small fresh basil leaves, to serve
salt and black pepper

FOR THE MARINARA SAUCE
1 large onion
3 garlic cloves
olive oil
1 cup red wine
1½ tbsp dried oregano
1 bay leaf
5 tbsp tomato paste
5 tbsp water
2 lb tomatoes
½ cup fresh basil leaves
½ tsp sugar
salt and black pepper

Preheat oven to 350°F | Line a baking sheet | Large deep frying pan with a lid over medium heat | Boiling water | Large saucepan | Food processor | Frying pan

To make the sauce, peel and finely chop the onion and garlic | Add some oil to the large frying pan and cook the onions for 7 minutes, stirring occasionally, until softened | Add the garlic and cook for another minute, until the smell of the garlic fills the room | Add the red wine and stir, then cook for 5 minutes until the wine is bubbling and starting to thicken | Add the oregano and bay leaf and stir | Add the tomato paste and water and stir again

Finely chop the tomatoes and scrape them into the pan with all the juices | Tear the basil leaves into the pan and stir everything together | Add the sugar and some salt and pepper to taste | Put the lid on the pan, reduce the heat to medium-low, and leave to simmer for 15–25 minutes, stirring occasionally (the longer you leave it, the richer the sauce) | Uncover and simmer for 10 minutes | When it's ready the sauce should be rich, luscious, and thick | Taste and adjust the seasoning if necessary

While the sauce is simmering, in the large saucepan, bring water to a boil and add a pinch of salt | Add the pasta and cook until al dente, according to the package directions | Drain and rinse the pasta under cold water for 30 seconds to cool it to room temperature

Tip the cold, cooked pasta into the food processor | Drain the black beans and the sun-dried tomatoes and add them to the food processor along with the chili powder and BBQ sauce | Blend to a thick paste, then pour the mixture into a large bowl

Place another frying pan over medium heat and add a little oil | Peel and finely chop the onion and 2 garlic cloves | Add the onion to the hot pan and cook for around 15 minutes, until soft | Add the garlic and stir it around until you've released the aroma (a minute or so) | Tip the onions and garlic into the bowl with the pasta and mix everything together | Add a little salt and pepper to taste

Wet your hands to stop the mixture sticking | Pull small pieces of the mixture out of the bowl and shape them into 1¼-inch balls | Arrange the balls on the lined baking sheet

Add a little olive oil to the pan you used to cook the onions and set over medium-high heat | When the pan is nice and hot, add the balls in batches, turning them over regularly until they brown all over, about 3–5 minutes | Transfer the browned pastaballs to the lined baking sheet and, once all the batches are done, transfer to the oven | Bake for 10 minutes

To serve, put a couple of large spoonfuls of the sauce into serving bowls and top each with 4 pastaballs | Garnish with a few torn-up basil leaves and a drizzle of olive oil | Serve immediately

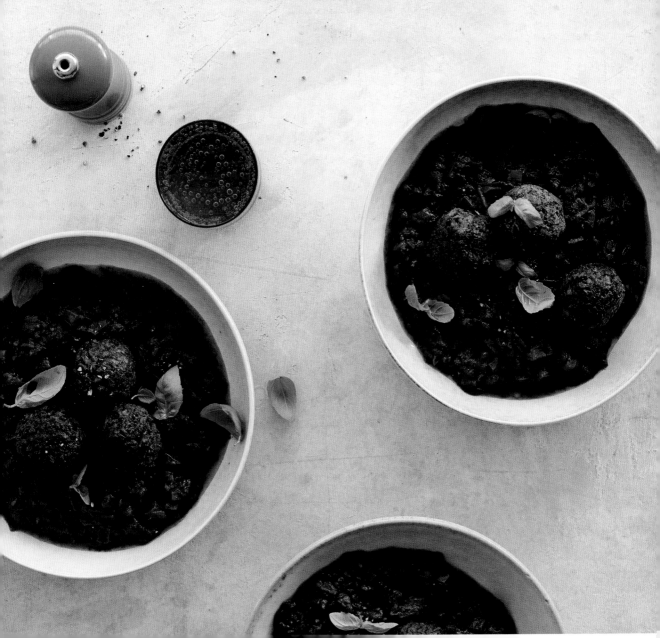

ROGAN BOSH!

This is our take on a Kashmiri specialty curry. It's meant to be red, rustic, and spicy. We've used our favorite vegetable—eggplant—and coconut yogurt to give the creamy texture, but you could use different veggies if you prefer. Serve with Naan (see page 203), Perfectly Boiled Rice (see page 207), or on its own for a lighter dish.

SERVES 2–4

4 garlic cloves
1½-inch piece fresh ginger
3 fresh red chilies
1 tbsp tomato paste
¼ cup water
1 large eggplant
3 tbsp vegetable oil
4 green cardamom pods
1 onion
6 black peppercorns
1 bay leaf
¼-inch cinnamon stick
1 tsp sugar
1 tsp ground cumin
2 tsp ground coriander
7 tbsp coconut yogurt
large pinch of garam masala
handful fresh cilantro, to serve
handful coconut flakes, to serve
salt

Blender | Large frying pan over medium-high heat | Large saucepan with a lid

Peel the garlic and ginger and put them into the blender | Rip the stems from 2 of the chilies, removing the seeds if you prefer a milder sauce, and add them to the blender | Add the tomato paste and ¼ cup water and blend to a smooth paste (add more water if needed)

Trim the eggplant and cut it into ⅓ x ¼-inch chunks | Add 2 tablespoons of the oil to the large frying pan | Add the eggplant and cook for about 10–15 minutes, turning regularly, until well browned on each side

While the eggplant is cooking, put the cardamom pods in a mortar and pestle and bash them to release the seeds (or use the end of a rolling pin) | Discard the shells | Peel and finely chop the onion

When the eggplant is browned, tip it onto a plate and set aside | Add the remaining oil to the pan along with the cardamom, peppercorns, bay leaf, and cinnamon and fry for 2 minutes | Add the chopped onion and sugar | Reduce the heat to medium and sauté for about 10–15 minutes, stirring the onions until they've softened (add a splash more oil to the pan if the onions begin to stick)

Add the ginger paste from the blender to the saucepan | Add the ground cumin and coriander and mix everything together well | Set the pan over medium-high heat and fry for 5 minutes, stirring regularly | Add the eggplant cubes and stir well | Add the coconut yogurt and stir it in (if it's too thick, add a little water to loosen—you want a thick, gravy-like consistency) | Cover with the lid and cook for 5 minutes

Rip the stem from the remaining chili, cut it in half lengthwise, and remove the seeds if you prefer a milder flavor, then slice finely | Taste the curry and season with salt or garam masala as necessary | Serve up onto bowls or plates, sprinkled with a little fresh cilantro, coconut flakes, and the finely sliced chili

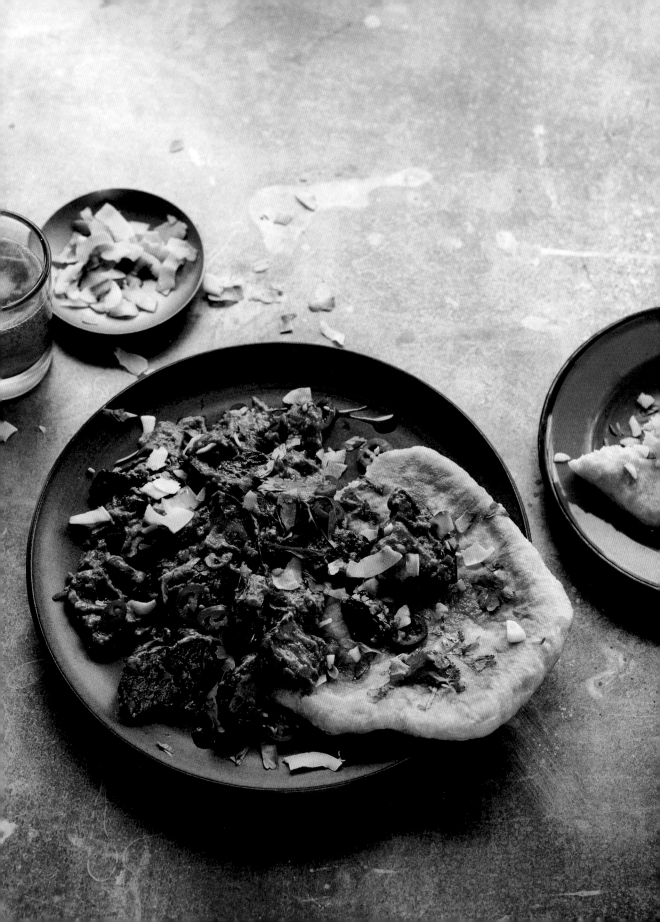

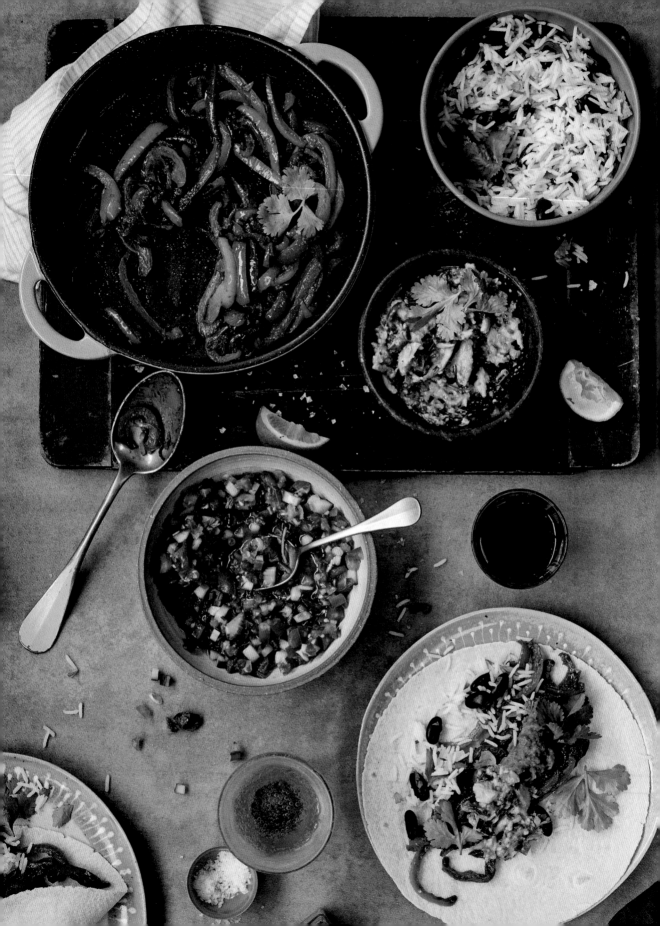

SWEET PEPPER FAJITAS

We challenged ourselves to create the ultimate healthy fajita and we think this combination of peppers, beans, guacamole, and salsa hits the spot. It's a delicious Spanish-inspired fried pepper recipe that works really well as part of a hybrid fajita platter that would please a crowd. It's great as a lunch, dinner, or even in a packed lunch!

MAKES 6 LARGE FAJITAS

olive oil, for frying
1 onion
2 garlic cloves
6 mixed red, yellow, and green bell
    peppers
½ tbsp dark brown sugar
1 tsp hot chili powder
1 tsp ground cumin
1 tsp paprika
¼ tsp cayenne pepper
¼ tsp garlic powder
a pinch of black pepper
1 can (15 oz) kidney beans
2 cups fresh cilantro leaves
1 can (15 oz) refried beans, optional
1 x portion Perfectly Boiled Rice
    (see page 207)
2 cups guacamole (store-bought
    or see page 194)
1 cup fresh salsa (store-bought or
    see page 195)
6 10-inch flour tortillas
3 limes
2 oz tortilla chips
salt and black pepper

Preheat the oven to 300°F | Large frying pan over medium heat

Add a little oil to the frying pan | Peel and finely slice the onion and garlic and add them to the pan | Cut the bell peppers in half, cut out the stems and seeds, slice the flesh into ¼-inch-wide strips, and add them to the pan | Sprinkle with the brown sugar and a pinch of salt

Put the chili powder into a small bowl with the cumin, paprika, cayenne pepper, garlic powder, and a pinch each of salt and pepper | Stir to mix and then tip over the peppers in the pan | Reduce the heat a little, then cook for 30 minutes until soft, stirring regularly so that the peppers don't stick to the pan

Meanwhile, drain the kidney beans and tip them into a serving bowl | Chop a third of the cilantro leaves and add them to the kidney beans | Spoon the refried beans, if using, into another bowl | Tip the cooked rice into another bowl | Spoon the guacamole and salsa into separate serving bowls

Put the tortillas on an ovenproof plate or baking sheet, cover with foil, and put in the oven to warm

The peppers are ready when they look well fried (but not blackened), are soft, and taste sweet and delicious | Transfer them to a serving bowl | Take the tortillas out of the oven and transfer them to a serving plate

Cut the limes into quarters | Roughly chop the remaining cilantro leaves | Fill a bowl with the tortilla chips

Take all the separate bowls to the table | Fill the fajitas with delicious dollops of everything and roll them up to enjoy!

THAI RED CURRY

Thai Red Curry may possibly be the best thing humans ever invented, at least since tools, the wheel, and (maybe) sliced bread. It's a feel-good meal with a hell of a kick. It's always best when you make your own paste; it doesn't take long and you can keep half for Tom Yum Soup (see page 63) or freeze it for later.

SERVES 4

1 red bell pepper
1 green bell pepper
1 fresh red chili
7 oz mushrooms
2 oz baby corn
2 tbsp vegetable oil
1 can (14 oz) coconut milk
⅔ cup vegetable stock
1 tbsp palm sugar (or regular sugar)
2 tbsp agave syrup
¼ cup soy sauce
6 oz baby plum tomatoes
2 oz snow peas
half a 15-oz can lychees, optional

FOR THE THAI RED CURRY PASTE
(MAKES ABOUT ¾ CUP)
1 tsp cumin seeds
2 tbsp coriander seeds
¾-inch piece fresh ginger
5 shallots
5 garlic cloves
2 lemongrass stalks
3 fresh red chilies
1 red bird's eye chili, optional
1 tsp black peppercorns
½ roasted red pepper from a jar
2 tbsp tomato paste
3 kaffir lime leaves
½ lime
5 sprigs fresh cilantro, plus extra
    for garnish
2 tsp salt
3 tbsp water

Blender | Large deep frying pan or wok over high heat

To make the Thai red curry paste, scatter the cumin and coriander seeds over the pan and toast for 2 minutes | Peel the ginger by scraping off the skin with a spoon and roughly chop | Peel and roughly chop the shallots | Peel the garlic | Trim and roughly chop the lemongrass | Rip the stems from the chilies, removing the seeds if you prefer a milder sauce

Put the toasted seeds into the blender along with the ginger, shallots, garlic, and lemongrass | Add the fresh red chilies, bird's eye chili, if using, peppercorns, roasted red pepper, tomato paste, and the lime leaves | Squeeze in the lime juice, catching any seeds in your other hand | Add the sprigs fresh cilantro, salt, and a splash of water, then whizz until really smooth with no bits, adding up to 3 tbsp of water to loosen it if necessary | Spoon ¼ cup of the paste into a bowl and set the rest aside to use another time (freeze it in batches of ¼ cup)

Cut the red and green bell peppers in half and cut out the stems and seeds, then cut into ¾-inch chunks | Rip the stems from 2 of the chilies, removing the seeds if you prefer a milder flavor, and cut into slices | Slice the mushrooms and halve the baby corn

Put the pan back over high heat and add the oil | When it's hot, add ¼ cup curry paste and fry for 2 minutes, until the paste deepens in color and smells amazing | Pour in the coconut milk and vegetable stock and stir well to mix everything together | Add the sugar, agave syrup, soy sauce, bell peppers, chili, mushroom, baby corn, tomatoes, and snow peas | Drain the lychees, if using, and add them to the pan | Bring to a boil and simmer for 7–10 minutes, until the vegetables are cooked through | Taste and adjust the seasoning, adding salt, sugar, or agave syrup as required

Spoon the curry into bowls, garnish with a handful of cilantro leaves, and serve alongside white rice

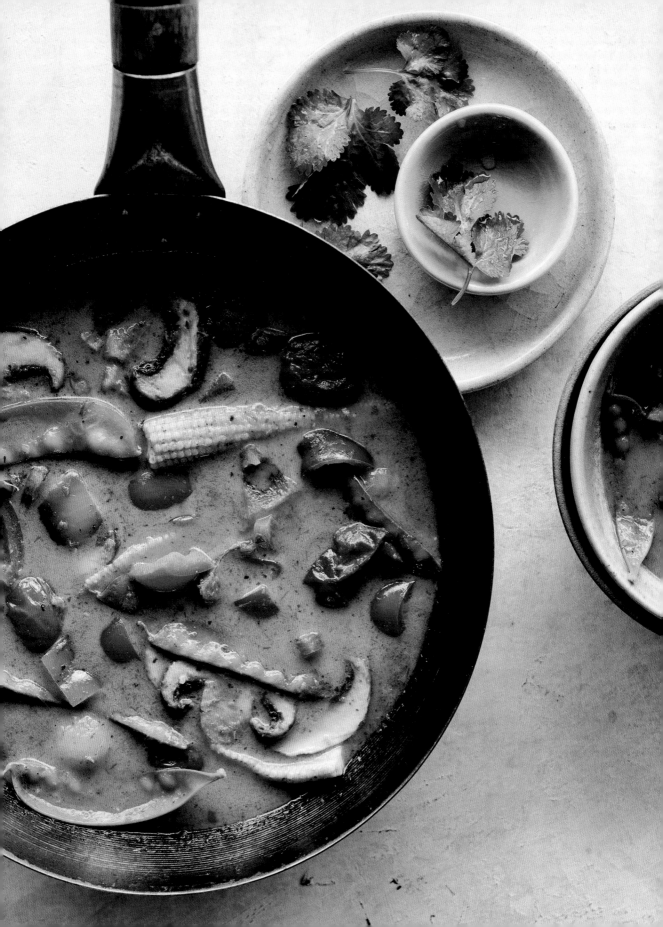

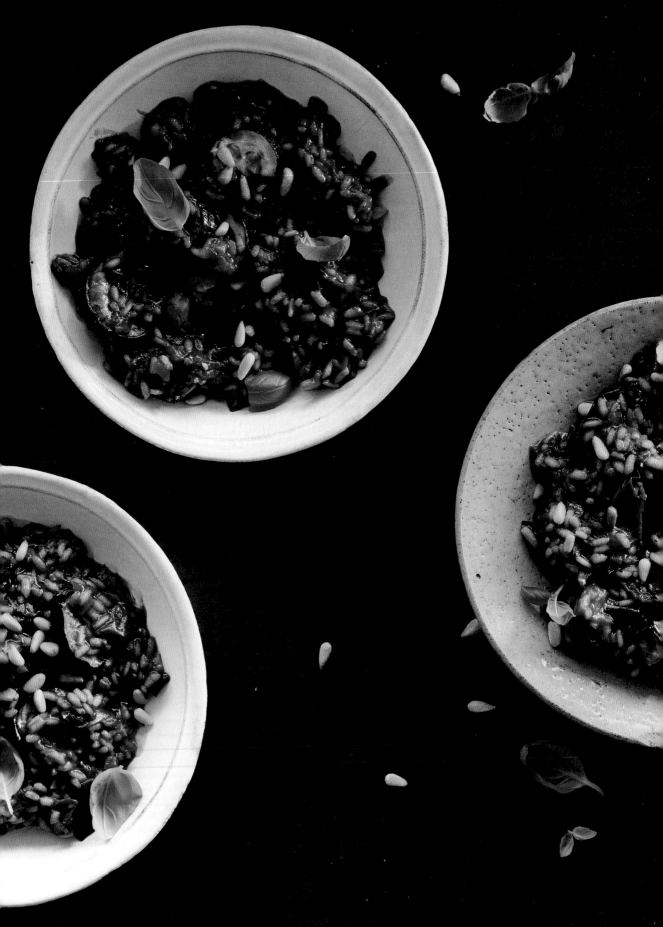

RED RATATOUILLE RISOTTO

Sometimes ideas hide in plain sight: we thought to ourselves, why couldn't we use red wine to make risotto? This controversial idea has upset some but pleased many more, with hundreds of people recreating this dish and sending us their pictures. It has all the goodness of risotto but with the romantic flair of red wine.

SERVES 4

1 eggplant (about 9 oz)
1 zucchini (about 7 oz)
6 tomatoes (about 1 lb)
¼ cup olive oil
1 large red onion
2 garlic cloves
5 sun-dried tomatoes in oil
2 sprigs fresh rosemary
2 sprigs fresh thyme
3¾ cups vegetable stock
2 tbsp tomato paste
1 cup + 2 tbsp risotto rice
½ cup red wine
1½ tbsp dairy-free butter or spread
2 tbsp pine nuts, to serve
handful fresh basil leaves, to serve
salt and black pepper

Preheat oven to 350°F | Line a baking sheet | Medium saucepan over low heat | Medium saucepan over medium heat

Trim the eggplant, zucchini, and tomatoes and cut them into 1-inch chunks | Put them all on the lined baking sheet, drizzle over 2 tablespoons of the oil, and season with salt and pepper | Put the pan in the oven and bake for 40 minutes

Meanwhile, peel and finely chop the red onion and garlic | Finely chop the sun-dried tomatoes | Remove the leaves from the herbs by running your thumb and forefinger from the top to the base of the stems (the leaves should easily come away), then finely chop

Place the stock in the medium saucepan over low heat and keep warm

Warm the remaining 2 tablespoons of oil in the other pan | Add the chopped red onion to the pan and cook until soft and translucent, about 10–15 minutes | Add the garlic and cook for 1 minute longer | Add the rosemary and thyme, sun-dried tomatoes, and tomato paste and give everything a stir | Cook for another 4–5 minutes

Pour the risotto rice into the pan and stir it around for 1 minute | Increase the heat slightly, pour in the red wine, and stir until the rice has absorbed all the wine | Now start adding the stock, a ladleful at a time, waiting until the stock has been absorbed before adding another ladleful (you might not need all of it)

After 15 minutes, the rice should be about 2–3 minutes away from being perfectly al dente | Take the roasted ratatouille vegetables out of the oven, scrape them into the pan, and fold them into the risotto along with all their juices | Stir until the rice is just cooked | Remove the pan from the heat and add the dairy-free butter | Season with salt and pepper

Divide among 4 bowls | Sprinkle with the pine nuts and garnish with fresh basil leaves

SAAG ALOO CURRY

This is definitely one of our healthier curries, but it's also powerfully spicy and tastes like takeout at home. There are lots of layers of flavor, the fenugreek being the star. We've made our spinach three ways to get maximum creaminess and freshness. Serve this with a couple of other curries for a DIY Indian sensation.

SERVES 2–4

FOR THE POTATOES
1 lb new potatoes
1 white onion
3 garlic cloves
2 tbsp sunflower oil
¼ tsp cumin seeds
1 tsp ground turmeric
2 tsp garam masala
½ tsp salt

FOR THE CURRY
1 white onion
1 fresh chili
2 garlic cloves
2⅓-inch piece fresh ginger
2 medium tomatoes (about 6 oz)
14 oz baby spinach
5 tbsp water
2 tbsp sunflower oil
2 tbsp garam masala
1 tsp ground turmeric
1 tbsp ground coriander
1 tsp ground fenugreek
1 tsp salt, plus a little extra
½ tsp sugar
7 tbsp soy cream
½ lemon

Medium saucepan of boiling salted water over high heat | Large frying pan over medium heat | Blender | Deep frying pan with a lid over medium heat

Peel the potatoes and cut them all in half | Put them into the medium saucepan and add just enough water to cover | Put the pan over high heat and bring to a boil, then immediately reduce the heat to medium and simmer until cooked, about 12–15 minutes | Take the pan off the heat and drain the potatoes in a colander

Meanwhile, peel and finely chop the onion | Peel and mince the garlic | Add the oil to the large frying pan over medium heat | Sprinkle in the cumin seeds and stir until they release their aroma, about 1 minute

Add the chopped onion and garlic and stir until the onion has softened, about 15 minutes | Add the potatoes, the turmeric, garam masala, and salt | Stir until the potatoes have taken on the color of the spices | Remove from the heat and set aside

Peel and finely dice the onion for the curry | Rip the stem from the chili, cut it in half lengthwise (remove the seeds for a milder sauce), then finely chop | Peel and mince the garlic | Peel the ginger by scraping off the skin with a spoon and finely chop | Finely chop the tomatoes

Roughly chop one-quarter of the spinach and finely chop another one-quarter | Put the remaining spinach into the blender with the water and whizz until completely blended

Add the oil to the deep-frying pan | Scrape in the chopped onions and garlic and fry until soft, about 10–15 minutes | Add the chili and ginger and stir for 2 more minutes | Add the tomatoes and stir until softened, about 3–5 minutes | Add the garam masala and turmeric, the ground coriander, fenugreek, salt, and sugar and stir until well combined

Add the roughly chopped spinach and stir until completely wilted | Add the finely chopped spinach and stir to mix | Pour in the blended spinach and stir until you have a dark green sauce | Simmer until thickened, about 10 minutes

Pour in the soy cream and stir in the potatoes | Cook until the sauce is bubbling slightly | Squeeze in the juice of the lemon, catching any seeds in your other hand | Serve hot alongside rice or naan

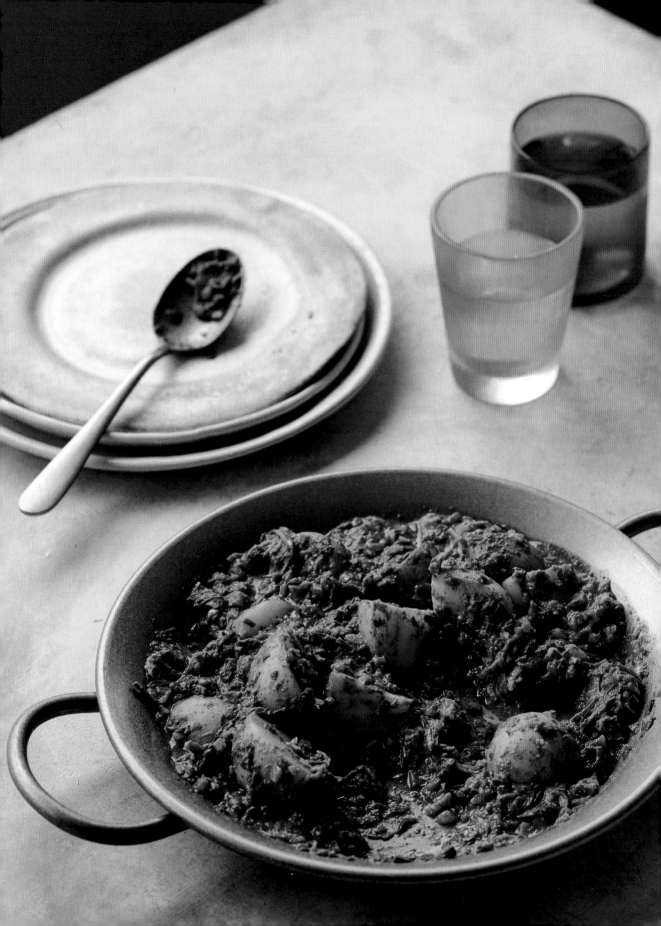

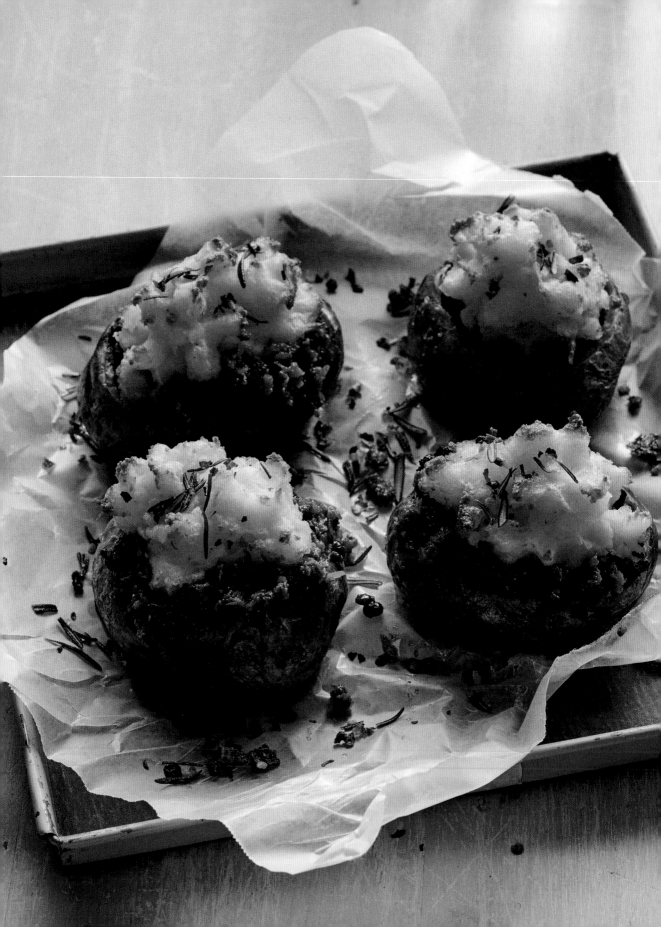

SHEPHERD'S POTATO

This is our (slightly ridiculous) remix of two British classics: shepherd's pie and jacket potato. We've turned them on their heads to create possibly the poshest jacket potato you will ever eat. The hearty, smoky filling and fluffy potato goodness create a night-in dish to impress.

MAKES 6

6 large baking potatoes
2 tbsp olive oil, plus a little bit extra
1 white onion
1 celery stalk
1 medium carrot
2 garlic cloves
3 sprigs fresh rosemary, plus extra
    to serve
3 sprigs fresh thyme
2 tsp whole-grain mustard
3 tbsp tomato paste
1 tbsp soy sauce
5 oz cremini mushrooms
4 oz cooked puy lentils (homemade
    or store-bought)
1 cup vegetable stock
1½ tbsp dairy-free butter or spread
2 tbsp nutritional yeast
1 tsp chili flakes, to serve
salt and black pepper

Preheat the oven to 390°F | Baking sheet | Deep frying pan over medium heat

Put the potatoes on the baking sheet and prick them with a fork | Drizzle with the 2 tablespoons of olive oil, season with salt and pepper, then rub them all over until completely covered | Put the pan in the hot oven and bake for 45–60 minutes, until soft

Peel and finely chop the white onion | Trim the leaves and root from the celery, then finely chop | Trim the carrot, peeling it if you like, and finely chop

Add a little oil to the hot pan | Add the chopped onions, celery, and carrots and fry until they start to soften, about 5–10 minutes | Peel and crush the garlic into the pan | Remove the leaves from the rosemary and thyme by running your thumb and forefinger from the top to the base of the stems (the leaves should easily come away), finely chop, and add to the pan | Season and cook for 2–3 minutes | Add the mustard, tomato paste, and soy sauce and stir | Reduce the heat to a light simmer

Chop the mushrooms very finely and add them to the pan | Add the lentils, stir everything together, and cook for 5–7 minutes | Pour in the stock and mix

When they're done, take the potatoes out of the oven (but leave the oven on) and let them cool down for a few minutes | Use a sharp knife to cut a round lid off the top of each potato | Scoop out the fluffy middles, leaving at least a ⅓-inch shell all round the insides, and transfer to a bowl | Add the dairy-free butter, nutritional yeast, and a pinch of salt and pepper to the bowl and mash

Fill each potato to the brim with the mushroom filling and top with a large dollop of mashed potato | Return the baking sheet to the oven and bake for 10–15 minutes to get the topping nice and crispy | Take the tray out of the oven | Sprinkle each potato with chili flakes, the remaining chopped rosemary, and some pepper before serving

SPAGHETTI BOLOGNESE

Our "spag bol" has all the deliciousness of the original, but with minced mushrooms providing the rich, smoky flavor. If you're looking for a warming, satisfying, and healthy(ish) dinner, then look no further. Perfect for a date night and great with a glass of red wine.

SERVES 4–6

1½ lb cremini mushrooms
1 tbsp olive oil
1 lb spaghetti
a few small fresh basil leaves, to serve
salt and pepper

FOR THE TOMATO SAUCE
2 red onions
1 celery stalk
4 garlic cloves
2 carrots
1 tbsp olive oil
1 tbsp tomato paste
1¼ cups red wine
1 tsp balsamic vinegar
½ tbsp dried oregano
1 bay leaf
2 tsp soy sauce

Food processor | Large frying pan over high heat | Large saucepan

Put the mushrooms in the food processor and pulse until very finely minced (you can chop them if you prefer, but it's quicker with a food processor)

Pour the oil into the frying pan | Add the mushrooms and season with a small pinch of salt and pepper | Cook for 10–15 minutes, stirring regularly, until all the liquid has evaporated and the mushrooms are well browned | Take the pan off the heat, transfer the mushrooms to a bowl, and set aside

Peel and roughly chop the onions for the tomato sauce | Trim the leaves and root from the celery and roughly chop | Peel the garlic | Trim the carrots and peel if the skin is tough, then roughly chop | Put the chopped vegetables and garlic into the food processor and mince well

Put the same pan back over medium-high heat and add the oil | Add the minced onions, garlic, carrots, and celery and cook for about 10 minutes, until all the vegetables are soft | Stir in the tomato paste | Add the red wine, balsamic vinegar, oregano, bay leaf, and soy sauce | Stir everything together and then turn down the heat | Simmer for 10 minutes

Meanwhile, bring a large saucepan of water to a boil over high heat and season with a big pinch of salt | Add the pasta to the pan and cook until al dente, according to the package directions | Spoon a scant ½ cup of the pasta water into a cup and set aside | Drain the pasta

Taste the sauce and season with salt and pepper | Add the minced mushrooms to the simmering sauce, turn up the heat, and pour in the reserved pasta water | Stir everything together and let the sauce simmer for another 3–5 minutes to warm through

Pour the sauce into the pasta pot and stir everything together so that the sauce completely covers the pasta | Scatter in the basil leaves and grind over some black pepper | Serve to happy faces!

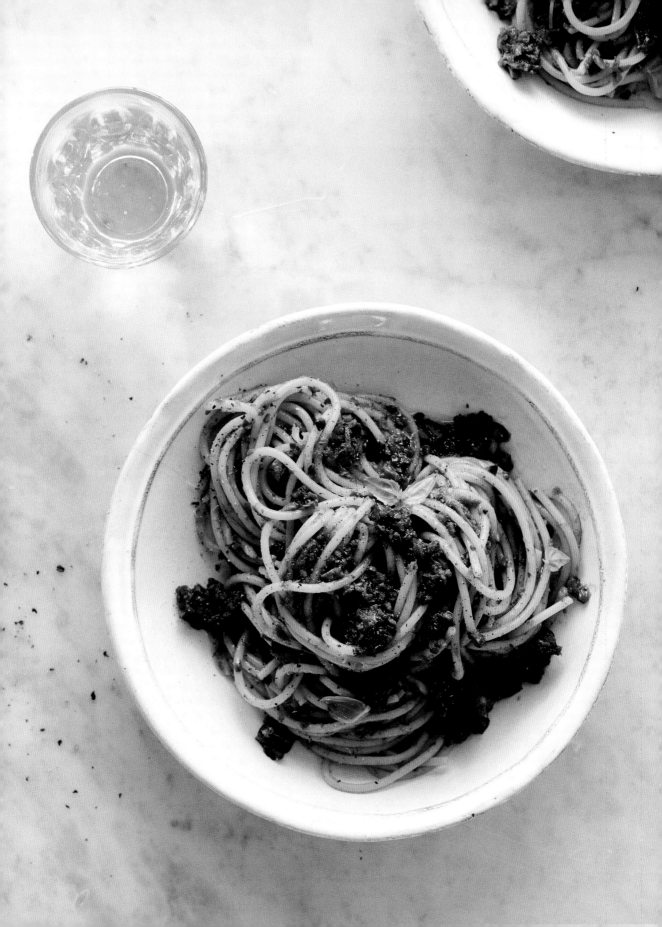

03

SHOW-PIECES

Now it's real wow time
Create awesome showpieces
To impress your guests

BURRITO SAMOSAS

This two-dish combination is a BOSH! classic and an internet sensation. This is the traditional burrito ingredients in an unfamiliar but fantastic form. It's perfect for lunch, dinner, or you can take it on the go with you. It's a hearty, full meal best served with salad and Guacamole (see page 194) or Salsa (see page 195).

MAKES 5

3 russet or other fluffy potatoes (about 1 lb)

1 red onion

3 garlic cloves

1 red bell pepper

1 fresh red chili

3 tbsp vegetable oil

2 tsp smoked paprika

1 tbsp ground coriander

2 tsp ground cumin

1 tbsp + ½ tsp Tabasco sauce, or to taste

1 can (15 oz) black beans

2 cups cooked basmati rice (store-bought or Perfectly Boiled Rice, see page 207)

1½ limes

1 cup fresh cilantro leaves

3½ oz dairy-free cheese

6 10-inch flour tortillas

guacamole (store-bought or see page 194), to serve

salsa (store-bought or see page 195), to serve

salt

Preheat oven to 350°F | Line a baking sheet | Medium saucepan over high heat | Large frying pan | Pastry brush

Peel the potatoes and chop them into ⅓-inch chunks | Put them into the medium saucepan and add just enough water to cover | Set the pan over high heat and bring to a boil, then immediately reduce the heat to medium and simmer until cooked, about 10 minutes | Take the pan off the heat and drain the potatoes in a colander

Meanwhile, peel and finely chop the red onion and garlic | Cut the bell pepper in half and cut out the stem and seeds, then finely chop | Rip the stem from the chili, cut it in half lengthwise, and remove the seeds if you prefer a milder flavor, then finely chop

Set the large frying pan over medium heat and add the vegetable oil | Once it's hot, add the minced vegetables and fry until soft, about 10 minutes | Add the smoked paprika, ground coriander, cumin, 1 tablespoon of the Tabasco, and a pinch of salt to the pan and stir everything together | Add the potatoes to the pan and stir until they've taken on all the colors and flavors and begun to crisp up slightly on the sides, about 10 minutes | Drain the black beans and tip them into the pan | Stir until warmed through | Take the pan off the heat and transfer the contents to a mixing bowl

Tip the cooked rice into a mixing bowl and fluff it with a fork | Cut the limes in half and squeeze in the juice, catching any seeds in your other hand | Scatter over the cilantro leaves, a pinch of salt, and ½ teaspoon of the Tabasco and stir them into the rice

Grate the dairy-free cheese into a bowl

Take one of the tortillas and cut into 5 equal-sized wedges | Cut across the curved edge of each wedge so that you have a straight-sided triangle | Set aside these triangles, which will be used to seal your samosas

90

Take another tortilla and lay it out on a clean work surface | Take about one-fifth of the rice and place it in the center of the tortilla | Follow with one-fifth of the dairy-free cheese and then one-fifth of the potato mixture | Shape the filling roughly into triangles with your hands, making sure it is in the middle of the tortilla | Place one of the tortilla triangles on top of the ingredients and press down slightly | Brush the rim of the round tortilla as well as the tortilla triangle with water (this will act as a glue to stick them together) | Fold the edges of the tortilla into the middle to form a triangle | Put the "samosa" on the lined baking sheet, fold side down | Repeat with the remaining samosas

Put the pan in the oven and bake for 20–25 minutes, until the samosas are crisp to the touch | Remove from the oven and serve with guacamole and salsa for happy dipping!

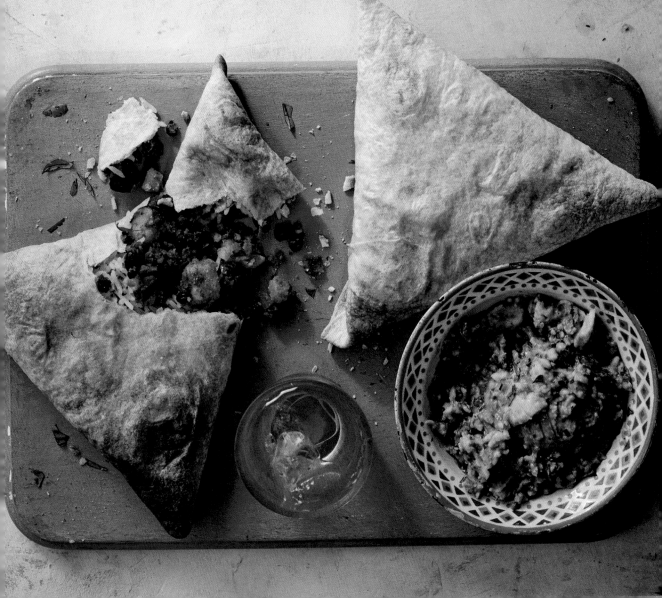

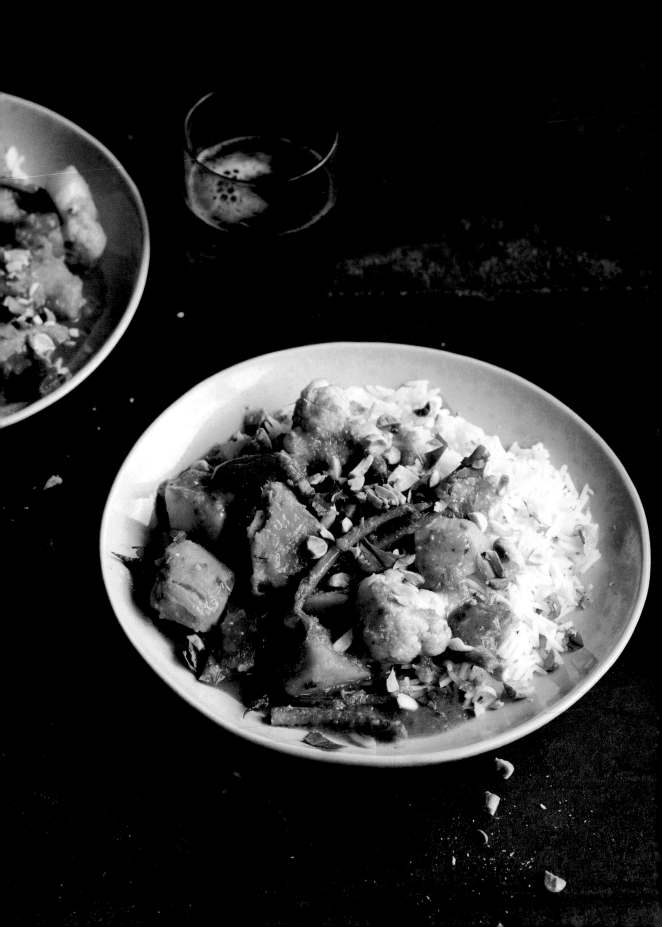

MASSAMAN CURRY

This is an absolute jaw-dropper of a curry. It has an incredible depth of hearty, umami flavor and a richness that keeps on giving. The spice kick is big but not too bold as it is infused throughout the dish. You could make this in the morning and leave it in the slow cooker all day for melt-in-your-mouth veggies. Serve with Perfectly Boiled Rice (see page 207).

SERVES 4

1 tsp fennel seeds
1 tsp cumin seeds
1 tsp coriander seeds
6 whole cloves
vegetable oil
2 lemongrass stalks
8 shallots
4 garlic cloves
1-inch piece fresh ginger
1 oz fresh cilantro sprigs
3 kaffir lime leaves
2 tbsp chili paste
1 can (14 oz) coconut milk
1 potato (about 8 oz)
2 sweet potatoes (about 1 lb)
1 red bell pepper
¼ lb green beans
½ small cauliflower
2 cups vegetable stock
1 tbsp tamarind paste
2 bay leaves
1 cinnamon stick
cooked rice, to serve
¼ cup roasted peanuts

Large saucepan over high heat | Blender

Put the fennel, cumin, and coriander seeds and cloves into the saucepan and toast for about 2 minutes, until fragrant | Transfer to the blender | Put the pan back on the heat and add a little oil

Trim the top and bottom off the lemongrass and carefully cut them in half lengthwise | Peel the shallots and garlic | Peel the ginger by scraping off the skin with a spoon | Separate the leaves and stems of the fresh cilantro and set both aside

Roughly chop the lemongrass, shallots, garlic, and ginger and tip them into the pan | Fry for 3 minutes, until lightly browned, then tip into the blender | Add the lime leaves, chili paste, and cilantro stems | Blend until you've created a completely smooth paste with a deep brown color and no bits | Pour back into the pan, turn the heat up to medium-high, and fry for 2 minutes, or until golden brown | Pour in the coconut milk, reduce the heat to medium, and let it bubble away slowly until reduced by a third

Meanwhile, peel the potato and sweet potatoes and chop into 1¼-inch cubes | Cut the bell pepper in half and cut out the stem and seeds, then chop into 1¼-inch squares | Cut the green beans into 1-inch pieces | Break the cauliflower into small florets

Add the vegetable stock to the pan, followed by the potato, sweet potato, cauliflower, bell pepper, and green beans | Add the tamarind paste, bay leaves, and cinnamon stick and bring to a boil, stirring continuously | Immediately reduce the heat to low and leave to simmer for 45–60 minutes, stirring occasionally, until you have a very thick, rich, curry consistency

Chop the reserved cilantro leaves | Serve the curry alongside boiled rice, scattered with the roasted peanuts and fresh cilantro

GIANT BURRITO CAKE

A giant burrito, wrapped up warm then baked in a frying pan = the most amazing sharing platter you ever had! Inspired by our good friends at Jungle Creations, this dish is incredibly easy and impressive. It's been cooked time and time again by our fans and is one of our finest food remixes to date. You can see this in all its flavor-packed glory on page 96.

SERVES 8–10

4 oz cherry tomatoes
3 scallions
1 tbsp olive oil
6–7 10-inch flour tortillas
10 slices dairy-free cheese
1 lime

FOR THE VEGETABLE FILLING
2 medium sweet potatoes (about 1 lb)
2 tbsp olive oil
½–1 tsp chili flakes
1 red onion
1 red bell pepper
1 yellow bell pepper
1 green bell pepper
1 tbsp olive oil
1 tsp garlic powder
1 tsp paprika
1½ tsp cayenne pepper
1 tsp onion powder
1 tsp ground cumin
salt and black pepper

FOR THE RICE FILLING
2 tbsp olive oil
5 scallions
3 garlic cloves
2 cups cooked basmati rice (store-bought or Perfectly Boiled Rice, see page 207)
1 can (15 oz) black beans
¼ tsp Tabasco sauce
salt
1 tbsp ground cumin
12 sprigs fresh cilantro

Preheat oven to 350°F | Line 2 baking sheets | Large ovenproof frying pan | Medium saucepan | Pastry brush

To make the vegetable filling, first cut the sweet potatoes into ¼-inch-thick slices | Lay them out on one of the lined baking sheets, drizzle them with 1 tablespoon olive oil, and sprinkle over the chili flakes and a good pinch each of salt and pepper | Mix everything around so that the potatoes are well coated | Put the pan into the hot oven and bake for 30 minutes, then remove the pan and set it aside

While the potatoes are in the oven, peel and finely slice the red onion | Cut the bell peppers in half and cut out the stems and seeds, then cut them into slices | Spread the onion and pepper slices over the second lined baking sheet and drizzle them with 1 tablespoon olive oil | Sprinkle with the garlic powder, paprika, cayenne pepper, onion powder, and ground cumin | Mix everything together and then put the pan into the oven below the potatoes to bake for 20 minutes, then remove the pan and set it aside

To prepare the rice filling, set the large frying pan over medium heat and add 2 tablespoons of olive oil | Trim and finely slice the scallions | Peel and finely slice the garlic | Put the sliced scallions and garlic into the pan and stir them around until you've released the aroma of the garlic; this should take about 2–3 minutes | Tip in the cooked rice | Drain the black beans and add them to the pan

Add the Tabasco sauce, a good pinch of salt, and ground cumin to the pan and stir everything together, then take the pan off the heat | Pick the leaves from the cilantro and add them to the pan, discarding the stems or using them for something else | Stir everything together again | Tip the contents of the pan into a large serving bowl and then clean the pan ready to use again

Trim and finely chop the cherry tomatoes | Trim the scallions and finely chop | Put the tomatoes and chopped scallions into small bowls so that they are ready when you build your giant burrito cake

Now you're ready to put it all together and assemble your cake | Brush the frying pan with 1 tablespoon olive oil to stop the burrito cake sticking | Now arrange four of the tortillas around the edges of the pan as if you are laying out the petals of a flower and draping each one over the edges of the pan (if you are using a really big frying pan you might need one more tortilla to make sure your burrito cake will be completely sealed) | Press a final tortilla into the center of the pan so that the bottom of the pan is completely covered and there are no gaps

Now you're going to fill your burrito cake | First spoon half the rice into the burrito base and spread it out evenly with the back of a wooden spoon | Place a layer of dairy-free cheese slices on top of the rice, followed by a layer of the sweet potato slices | Next, take half the onion and pepper slices and place them on top of the sweet potato to make an even layer | Sprinkle over half the chopped cherry tomatoes and half the sliced scallions | Cut the lime in half and squeeze in the juice of one half, catching any seeds in the other hand | Repeat with a layer of rice, dairy-free cheese slices, sweet potato slices, onion and pepper slices, cherry tomatoes, scallions, and the juice from the other half of the lime so that you use up all of the ingredients | Make sure the filling is nice and even and as round as possible as this will form the shape of your burrito cake

Lay the remaining tortilla over the top of the filling to form a lid | Use a pastry brush or your finger to wet the edges of each tortilla with a thin coating of water (this will act as a glue to stick the tortillas together and seal the cake) | Fold the overhanging tortillas neatly over the filling and into the middle of the cake, starting with one tortilla and working your way around the cake, and smooth them down to seal the cake

Put the pan into the hot oven and bake the burrito cake for 20 minutes, until the filling is cooked through, the tortilla casing is golden, and the cake looks nice and solid | Take the pan out of the oven

To serve your burrito cake, place a large serving board on top of the pan and very carefully flip both the pan and board over to release the cake | Use a sharp knife to cut it into neat wedges and enjoy your giant burrito cake!

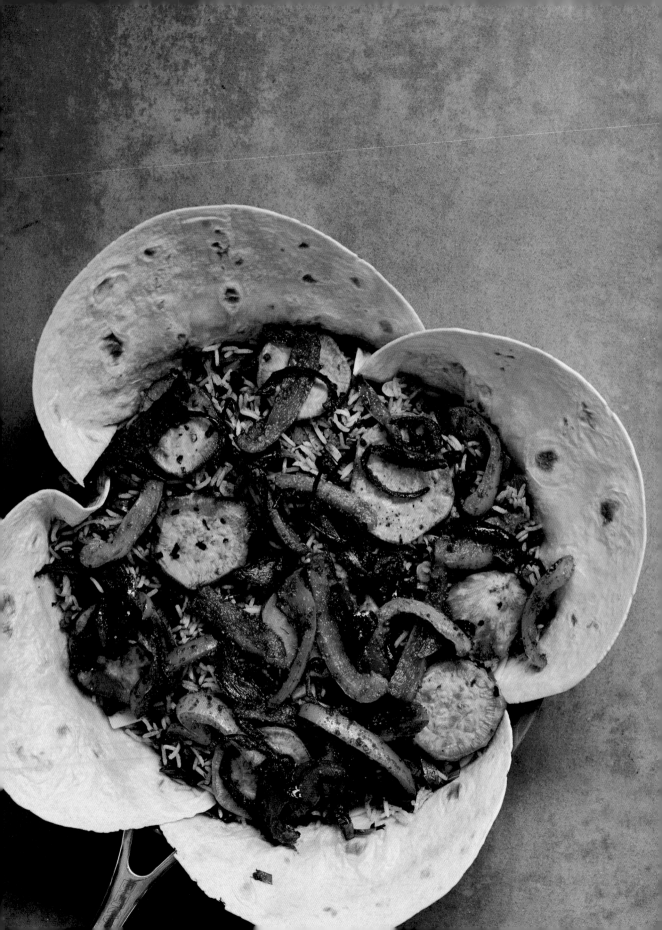

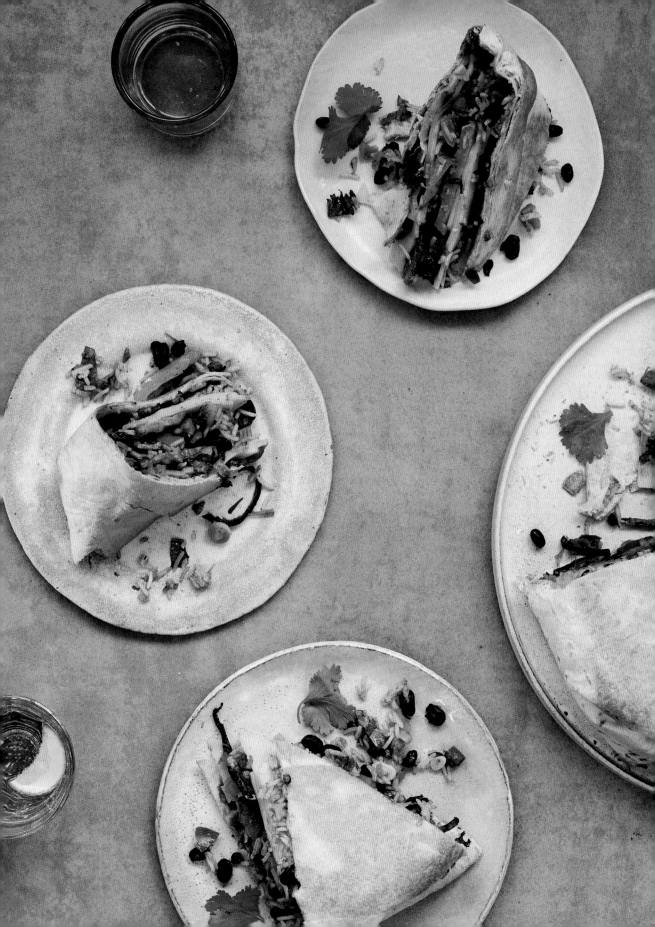

MEZZE CAKE

This is one of the finest dishes we've ever made or eaten, with every mouthful the perfect combination of flavors you could hope to get in a Middle Eastern restaurant. It's a proud remix of an entire cuisine into a cake and, while it is a bit of a labor of love, it's guaranteed to excite your taste buds. Check out the photo on page 100 for inspiration!

SERVES 8–10

2 eggplants

2 zucchini

olive oil

1 thin flatbread (under ¼ inch)

1¼ cups hummus (store-bought or see page 199)

2–3 tbsp sriracha

18–20 sun-dried tomatoes

7 tbsp olive tapenade (store-bought or see page 192)

2 cups cooked basmati rice (store-bought or Perfectly Boiled Rice, see page 207)

7 roasted red peppers from a jar

8 artichokes from a jar

7 tbsp baba ganoush (store-bought or see page 193)

FOR THE FALAFEL MIX

1 can (15 oz) chickpeas

1 small red onion

1 cup fresh parsley leaves

⅔ cup fresh cilantro leaves

2 tsp garlic powder

1½–2 tsp ground cumin

1½–2 tsp ground coriander

2 tsp harissa paste

2 tbsp all-purpose flour

1 tbsp olive oil

salt

Preheat oven to 350°F | Baking sheet drizzled with olive oil | 8-inch springform pan | Food processor | Grill pan

Cut off the stem ends of the eggplants and cut the flesh into slices about ¼ inch thick | Trim the zucchini and cut them into ¼-inch-thick slices | Set aside three of the nicest looking slices of each (choose ones that are roughly the same size) | Spread the rest over the greased baking sheet and drizzle them with a bit more oil | Rub the oil into the slices | Put the pan into the hot oven and roast for 30 minutes, until the vegetables are soft | Remove the pan from the oven and set it aside to cool

Next, place the flatbread on a cutting board and lay the springform pan on top of it | Cut around the pan with a sharp knife to make a flatbread round that will fit inside the bottom of it | Put the flatbread inside the pan and spread it with a ⅓-inch layer of hummus | Drizzle a tablespoon of chili sauce over the top of the hummus

You're now going to layer up the ingredients inside the pan to build up your mezze cake | First place a flat ring of sun-dried tomatoes all around the edge of the pan | Then, inside the ring of tomatoes, build another ring of roasted zucchini slices, placing one in the center if there is space | Fill in any gaps between the slices with spoonfuls of the olive tapenade

Next, spoon a layer of the cooked rice over the vegetables so that it is about ¼ inch deep all over and press it down firmly with the back of the spoon to get it nice and firm and even all over | Place a layer of the roasted eggplant and zucchini slices over the top of the rice layer and fill the gaps with more blobs of the olive tapenade | Once again, press down all over the top of the cake with a spoon to keep it all nice and compact (this step is important as it will hold the cake together when it cooks and ensure you get immaculate slices)

Cut the roasted peppers into ¾-inch strips and arrange them in a star shape over the top of the cake and fill the spaces in between the star with pieces of artichoke | Firm everything down again with the back of a spoon | Arrange more of the roasted zucchini around the edge of the pan and place some sun-dried tomatoes in the space in the middle | Fill in the gaps with spoonfuls of the baba ganoush

Next prepare the falafel topping | Drain the chickpeas and tip them into the food processor | Peel the onion and roughly chop it, then add it to the chickpeas | Throw in the fresh parsley and cilantro leaves, the garlic powder, the ground cumin, ground coriander, and the harissa paste | Spoon the flour into the food processor with the tablespoon of olive oil and pinch of salt | Whizz everything together until you have a thick paste | Spoon the falafel mixture all over the top of the cake and smooth it out using the back of the spoon or a frosting spatula as if you were icing a cake, until you have an even ⅓-inch layer

Put the cake in the hot oven and bake for 20–25 minutes, until the falafel on the top has hardened and everything is cooked through

While the cake is cooking, set the grill pan over medium-high heat and drizzle it with some olive oil | Heat the oil until it's really hot | Put the reserved slices of eggplant and zucchini into the hot pan and cook them on one side until they have defined char lines and are softened, then flip them over to cook the other side (try not to move them around too much in the pan as we want to make nice neat black grill marks); the eggplant will take around 5 minutes per side and the zucchini will take about 3–4 minutes per side | Remove the pan from the heat and transfer the slices to a plate

When the cake is ready, take it out of the oven | To finish and decorate it, spoon the remaining hummus on top and spread it out neatly until you have a ¼–⅓-inch layer all over the top of the cake | Now make it look pretty by decorating it with the grilled eggplant and zucchini slices and then drizzling it all over the top with the rest of the chili sauce | Finally, scatter over the fresh cilantro leaves

Carefully release the cake from the pan and reveal your masterpiece | You'll need to use a very sharp knife to slice the cake and serve it immediately | If the knife gets caught at any point, a sharp pair of scissors can help you to cut it more neatly | Make sure the flatbread at the bottom is completely cut through before you remove the slice so that everything comes out in one perfect tidy piece!

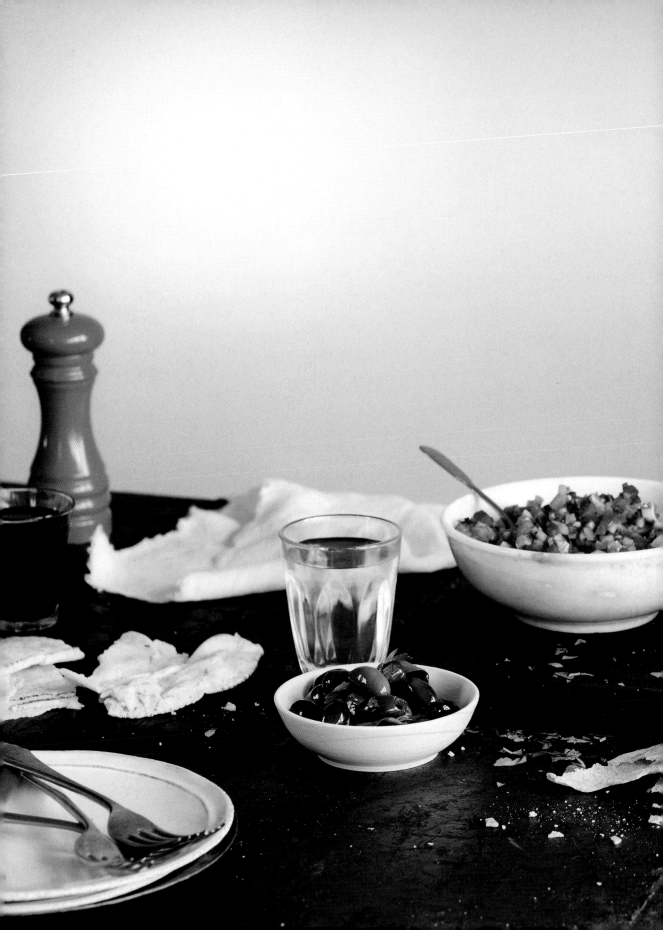

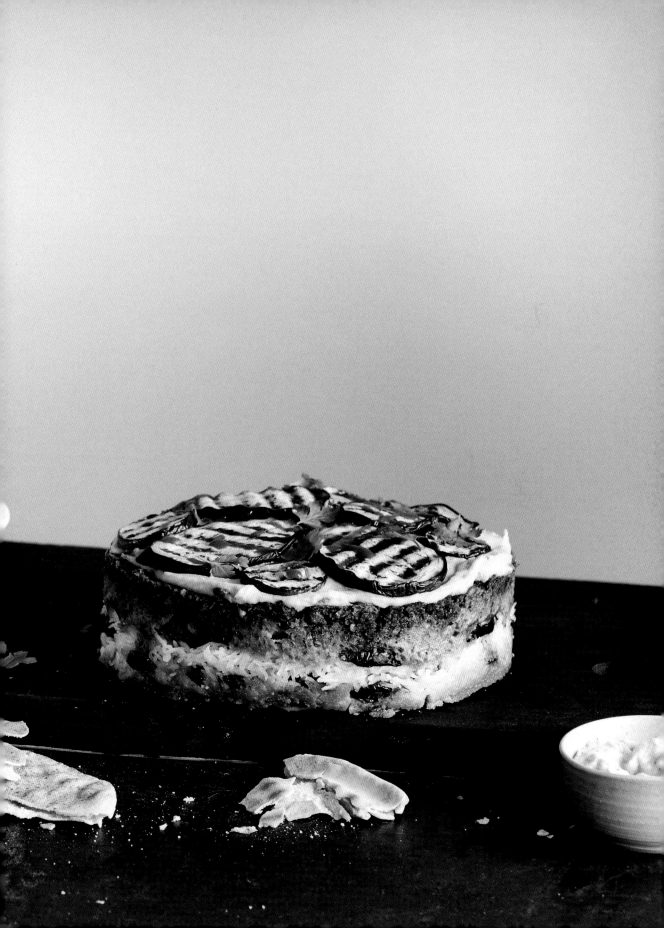

ULTIMATE CHILI

This deep, dark, and smoky chili is perhaps the richest we've tasted. The flavor comes from the mushroom base, but is boosted by untraditional ingredients like soy sauce, balsamic vinegar, maple syrup, and chocolate. You should absolutely leave it bubbling away if you have the time. It's so, so good—you'll be bowled over by the end result. Turn the page for a mouthwatering preview.

SERVES 6

14 oz mushrooms
olive oil
¼ tsp salt
¼ tsp black pepper
2 red onions
4 garlic cloves
2 fresh red chilies
14 sprigs fresh cilantro
1 celery stalk
1 red bell pepper
1 tbsp tomato paste
1 cup red wine
2 tsp soy sauce
1 tsp balsamic vinegar
2 cans (14.5 oz each) chopped tomatoes
1 can (15 oz) black beans
1 can (15 oz) kidney beans
1½ tsp maple syrup
½ oz dark chocolate

FOR THE SPICE MIX
1 tsp chili powder
1 tsp ground cumin
1 tsp smoked paprika
½ tsp ground cinnamon
½ tsp dried oregano
½ tsp salt
½ tsp black pepper
1 bay leaf

Food processor | Frying pan over medium-high heat | Large saucepan over medium heat

Put the mushrooms in the food processor and pulse until very finely minced (you can chop them if you prefer, but it's quicker and better with a food processor)

Pour a little oil into the hot frying pan | Once the oil is hot, tip in the mushrooms with the salt and pepper and cook for 5 minutes | Take the pan off the heat, transfer the mushrooms to a bowl, and set aside

Peel and mince the red onions | Peel and mince the garlic | Rip the stems from the chilies, cut them in half lengthwise, and remove the seeds if you prefer a milder sauce, then chop finely | Remove the leaves from the cilantro and set aside | Finely chop the stems | Trim the leaves and root from the celery | Cut the bell pepper in half and cut out the stem and seeds | Cut the celery and pepper into very small chunks

Add a little oil to the large saucepan | Once it is hot, add the minced onions and garlic, the finely chopped cilantro stems, and the chilies and cook gently for 5–10 minutes, making sure you stir constantly | Add the chopped celery and bell pepper chunks to the pan and stir

Add all the spice mix ingredients to the pan and stir so that the spices are well mixed and coat all the vegetables | Stir in the tomato paste to give a rich color and depth of flavor | Pour the red wine, soy sauce, and balsamic vinegar into the pan and turn up the heat to high | Stir constantly until the liquid has reduced by two-thirds and the alcoholic aroma has subsided | Tip the chopped tomatoes into the pan, stir into the chili, and simmer for 5 minutes, until the sauce is noticeably thicker

Drain the black beans and kidney beans and add them to the pan along with the maple syrup, dark chocolate, and the minced mushrooms | Stir everything together really well and then reduce the heat to a very gentle simmer | Leave this bubbling away with the lid off, stirring occasionally until it's reduced to the right thickness (at least 10 minutes) | You can leave it bubbling for longer to deepen the flavors, adding more water if needed to keep the right consistency

Take the lid off the pan and remove the bay leaf | Stir the cilantro leaves into the chili and serve—or make Big Bad Nachos!

BIG BAD NACHOS

Shortly after the first chili came the first nachos. We're massive chili fans, but we always have loads left over and these nachos are a brilliant way to use it up. This dish is a sure-fire movie night crowd-pleaser. Feel free to adjust the quantities and experiment with soy cream, coconut yogurt, fresh chilies, or refried beans—see overleaf for serving inspiration.

SERVES 8

2 bags (7 oz each) tortilla chips
1 jar (7 oz) pickled jalapeños
1¾ oz dairy-free cheese such as our Garlic & Herb Cashew Cheese (see page 210), optional
1 cup Ultimate Chili (see opposite) or leftovers from a previous meal
¾ cup guacamole (store-bought or see page 194)
¾ cup fresh salsa (store-bought or see page 195)
handful fresh cilantro leaves

Preheat oven to 390°F | Large ovenproof dish (about 12 x 9-inch)

Tip the tortilla chips into the ovenproof dish so that they cover the bottom | Slice the jalapeños and scatter them over the tortilla chips | Throw in the dairy-free cheese, if using | Cover with the Ultimate Chili

Put the dish in the oven and bake until the tortilla chips have started to brown and the chili is heated through, about 10–15 minutes | Take the dish out of the oven

Dot random spots of guacamole and salsa over the top | Chop up the cilantro leaves and scatter them over the nachos

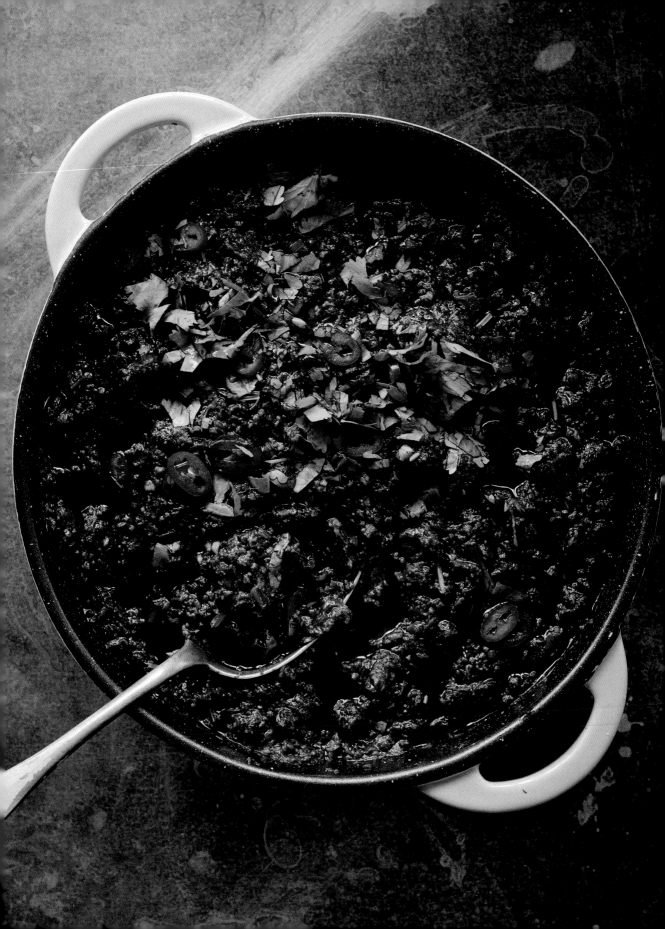

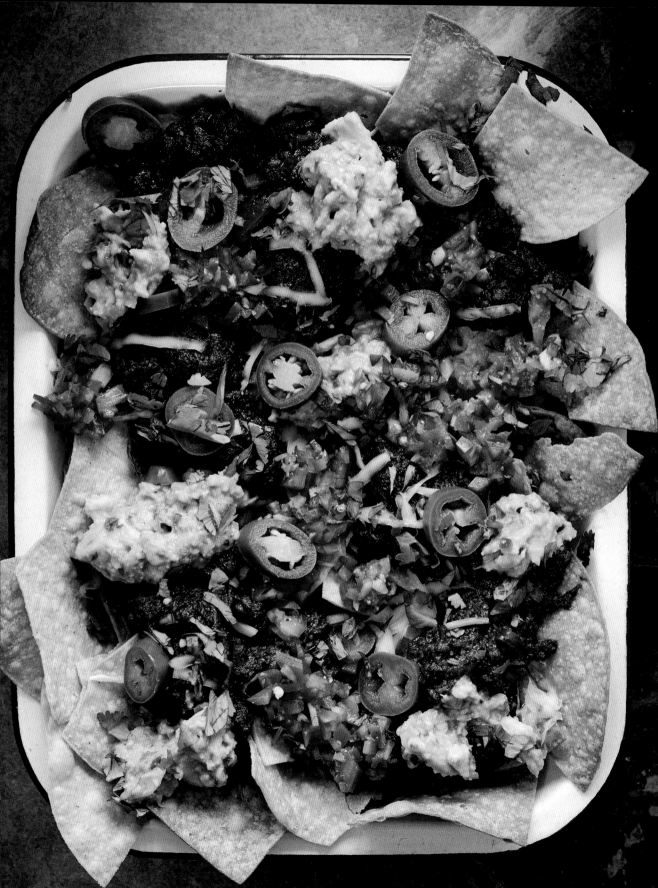

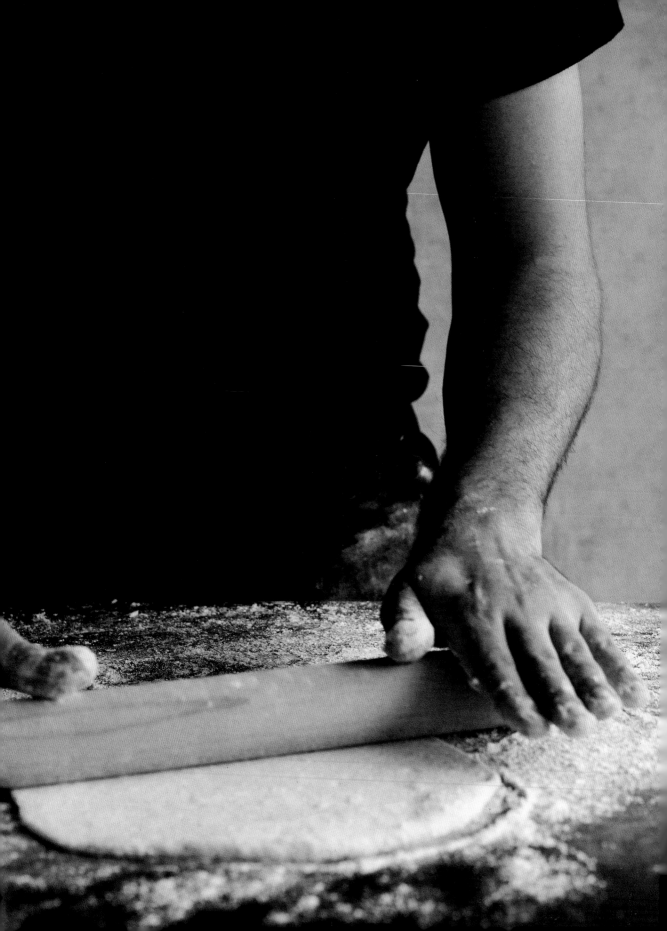

PERFECT PIZZA

Pizza, pizza. The perfect sharing food. It's satisfying, filling, and can be a healthy(ish) choice when it's done right. People are often afraid of dough-making but it doesn't take long and the kneading is incredibly satisfying, maybe even meditative. Make double and you can freeze half for next time. We recommend a pizza stone for a really good crust.

BASIC PIZZA DOUGH

MAKES 2 LARGE PIZZA CRUSTS

3²/₃ cups bread flour
½ envelope (1⅛ tsp) fast-acting dry
   yeast
1½ tsp salt
1 cup + 7 tbsp water, at room
   temperature

Clean work surface dusted liberally with flour

Measure the flour into a large bowl | Stir in the yeast and salt and mix it all together well | Use your hands to make a well in the middle of the bowl | Pour in the water and slowly mix together, kneading well with your fingers | When a dough has come together, bring it out of the bowl and put it on the floured work surface | Knead for 15 minutes, stretching and folding the dough, turning it 90 degrees, and then repeating until it becomes really smooth and springy | Wipe any flour or dough out of the bowl and rub the inside lightly with oil | Put the dough back in, cover with plastic wrap, and leave to rise for about 1 hour until doubled in size

Tip the risen dough back onto the work surface and give it another 60 seconds of kneading, then divide it into two | Cover each half with plastic wrap and leave to rise for another 30 minutes | You can store the dough in plastic wrap in the freezer for up to 1 month, defrosting completely before using

MIDDLE EAST PIZZA

With its Middle Eastern vibes, this pizza is a clear winner on pizza night. Feel free to play around with the ingredients. We use lots of jarred ingredients so it's a great pantry standby. Serve alongside hummus, tapenade, and any other mezze dishes you can think of!

MAKES 2 LARGE PIZZAS

flour, for dusting
Basic Pizza Dough (see page 107)
semolina, for dusting
4 artichoke hearts preserved in oil (from a jar)
1 red pepper preserved in oil (from a jar)
6 cherry tomatoes
6 sun-dried tomatoes
½ red onion
5 tbsp hummus (store-bought or see page 199), plus extra to serve
generous 3 tbsp olive tapenade (store-bought or see page 192), plus extra to serve
handful fresh cilantro, to serve
hot sauce, to serve

FOR THE TOMATO SAUCE
1 garlic clove
small handful fresh basil or 1 tsp dried
1 tbsp olive oil
¾ cup canned chopped tomatoes
1 tsp red wine vinegar

Preheat oven to 480°F | Pizza stone or heavy baking sheet heating up in the oven | Baking sheet dusted liberally with semolina | Clean work surface dusted liberally with flour | Blender | Rolling pin (or use a clean, dry wine bottle)

First make the tomato sauce | Peel the garlic clove and add it to the blender with the basil | Add the olive oil, canned tomatoes, and red wine vinegar | Whizz until really smooth

Tip one of the dough balls onto the floured work surface and roll it out to about 12-inch diameter | Carefully transfer to the baking sheet, laying it over the semolina | Spoon a thin layer of tomato sauce over the top of the pizza, spreading it all the way to the edges | Set aside

Take your artichoke hearts out of the jar and cut them in half | Take the pepper out of the jar and wipe off any excess oil, then cut into thin strips | Halve the cherry tomatoes and sun-dried tomatoes | Peel and finely slice the onion

Decorate your pizza crust with half the vegetables you've just prepared, making sure you leave a little space around them | Slide the crust onto the hot pizza stone or baking sheet in the oven and bake for 10 minutes | Meanwhile prepare the second pizza

Remove the cooked pizza from the oven and spoon about 8 small dollops each of hummus and tapenade around the pizza, as artfully as you can | Chop the cilantro leaves and sprinkle over the top, then splash with a few drops of hot sauce | Repeat with the second pizza and serve

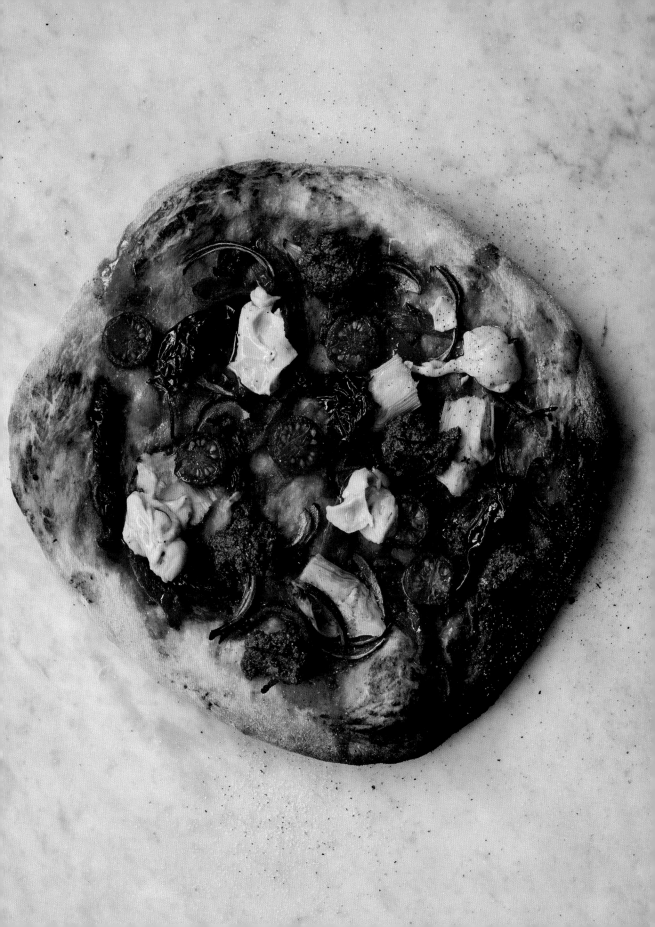

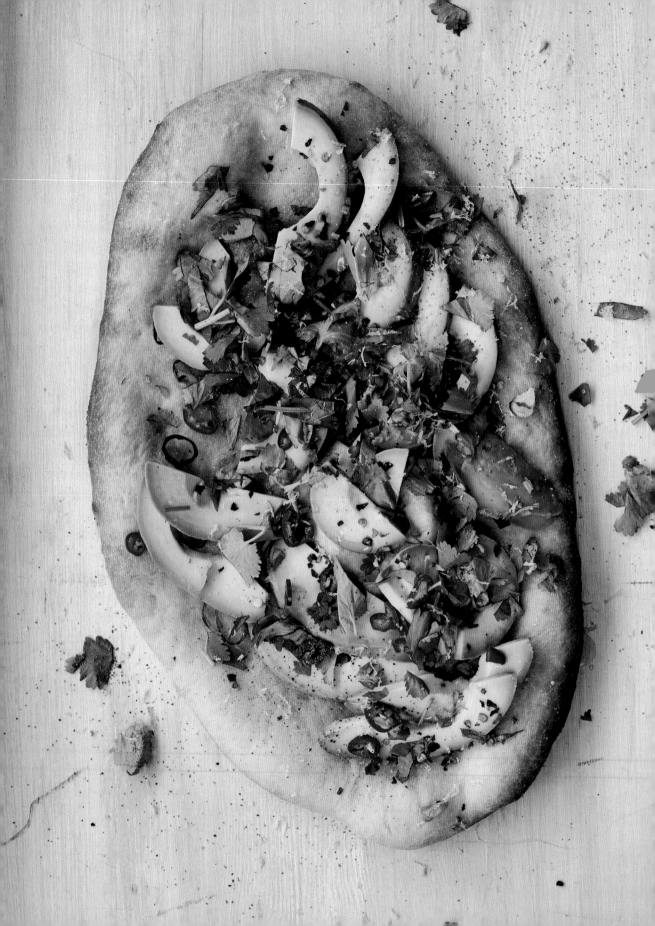

AVOCADO TOAST PIZZA

This is the ultimate hipster dish and works as a brunch as much as a main. Think of a really good garlic bread pizza with a big power-up of avocado and delicious cilantro and lemon zest.

MAKES 2 LARGE PIZZAS

1 garlic clove
1 fresh red chili
½ cup fresh cilantro
flour, for dusting
Basic Pizza Dough (see page 107)
semolina, for dusting
3 tbsp olive oil
6 avocados
1 lemon
1–2 tsp chili flakes
salt and black pepper
tomato salsa, for dipping, optional

Preheat oven to 480°F | Pizza stone or heavy baking sheet heating up in the oven | Rolling pin (or use a clean, dry wine bottle) | Baking sheet dusted liberally with semolina | Pastry brush

Peel and finely chop the garlic | Rip the stem from the chili, cut it in half lengthwise, remove the seeds if you prefer a milder flavor, and finely chop | Cut the stems from the cilantro and finely chop, reserving the leaves

Dust a clean, dry work surface liberally with flour | Roll out one of the dough balls to about 12-inch diameter | Carefully transfer to the baking sheet, laying it over the semolina | Brush the top of the pizza with half the olive oil | Sprinkle half the garlic, chili, and chopped cilantro stems all over the pizza crust | Carefully slide the pizza onto the hot pizza stone or baking sheet in the oven and cook for 10 minutes | Meanwhile, prepare the second pizza

Next prep the toppings | Halve and carefully pit the avocados by tapping the pit firmly with the heel of a knife so that it lodges in the pits, then twist and remove the pits | Run a spoon around the inside of the skin to scoop out the avocado halves, then slice them finely, keeping the shape of the avocado halves

Slide the cooked pizza crust onto a cutting board and put the second pizza in the oven

You're going to use 3 avocados for the first crust | Pick up the first half of slices and lay it on the pizza, then press down gently to fan out the slices neatly | Repeat until the pizza is almost completely covered in avocado | Halve the lemon and squeeze one half all over the pizza, catching any seeds in your other hand | Finely chop the cilantro leaves and scatter half over the pizza | Season with salt and black pepper and sprinkle with chili flakes

Remove the second pizza from the oven and repeat with the remaining toppings | Serve the pizzas on their own or with a tomato salsa for dipping, if using

JERK JACKFRUIT & PLANTAIN PIZZA

This evolved from our Reggae Reggae Pizza. We decided to badboy it up with spicy jerk jackfruit offset by sweet plantain. It's got a satisfying bite and comes fully loaded—this is a HOT pizza. Adjust the chilies to taste and add BBQ or jerk sauce for dipping.

MAKES 2 LARGE PIZZAS

Basic Pizza Dough (see page 107)
flour, for dusting
semolina, for dusting
2 tbsp olive oil
1 can (14 oz) young green jackfruit in spring water
1 ripe plantain (the skin should be more black than yellow)
BBQ or jerk sauce, to serve, optional

FOR THE JERK SAUCE
1 fresh Scotch bonnet chili
2 garlic cloves
5–7 sprigs fresh thyme
1 tsp ground cloves
1 tsp ground cinnamon
1 tsp ground nutmeg
2 tsp ground allspice
black pepper
olive oil

FOR THE TOMATO SAUCE
¾ cup canned chopped tomatoes
handful fresh basil or 1 tsp dried
1 garlic clove
1 tbsp olive oil
1 tsp red wine vinegar

Preheat oven to 480°F | Pizza stone or heavy baking sheet heating up in the oven | Blender | Rolling pin (or use a clean, dry wine bottle) | Baking sheet dusted liberally with semolina | Large frying pan

First make the jerk sauce by ripping the stem from the chili, cutting it in half lengthwise, and removing the seeds if you prefer a milder sauce, then finely chop | Peel and mince the garlic | Remove the leaves from the thyme by running your thumb and forefinger from the top to the base of the stems (the leaves should easily come away) and finely chop | Put the chili, garlic, thyme, cloves, cinnamon, nutmeg, and allspice in a mixing bowl with some black pepper and a dash of olive oil | Mix well

Take 1 tablespoon of the jerk sauce and put it into the blender with the ingredients for the tomato sauce | Whizz until really smooth

Dust a clean, dry work surface liberally with flour | Roll out one of the dough balls to about 12-inch diameter | Carefully transfer to the baking sheet, laying it over the semolina | Spoon a thin layer of tomato sauce over the top, spreading it all the way to the edges | Set aside

Put 1 tablespoon of oil into the frying pan and set it over medium heat | Drain the jackfruit and cut into thin slices, following the grain of the fruit from the bottom to the top | Add to the jerk marinade and stir to coat | You can leave to marinate for an hour for a deeper flavor, or add straight to the hot pan and fry for 5 minutes, stirring regularly | Remove from the heat and transfer half the fruit to the pizza

Put the remaining oil into the pan and put it back on the heat | Peel and finely slice the plantain | Add to the pan and sauté for 3–5 minutes, turning a couple of times, until golden brown | Take off the heat and add half the slices to the pizza

Carefully slide the pizza onto the hot pizza stone or baking sheet and cook for 10 minutes | Meanwhile, assemble the second pizza

Remove the cooked pizza from the oven and follow with the second | Serve with BBQ or jerk sauce, if using

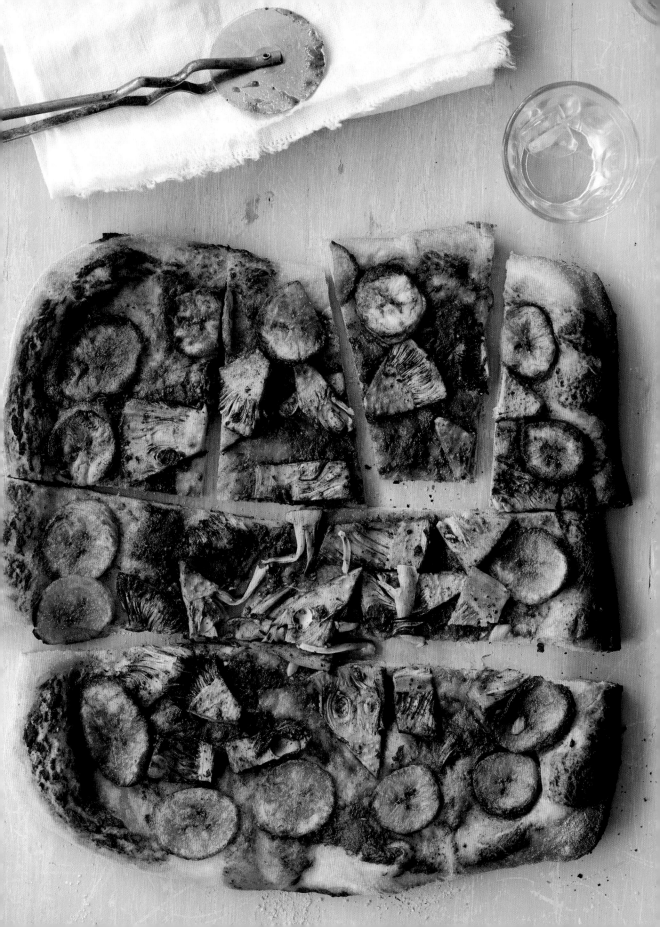

PETTIGREW'S PAELLA

This Spanish classic is loved by many, mastered by few. However, Henry's father has made a good effort and passed the recipe down proudly from father to son. Paella should never be stirred—unlike risotto, the rice needs to stay firm and not sticky. The lemon wedges served on every plate to be squeezed over before eating are absolutely nonnegotiable! Turn the page to see this in all its glory.

SERVES 4–6

1 large red bell pepper
¾ cup butter beans or lima beans
1 small onion
1 large garlic clove
1 medium tomato (about 4 oz)
5 oz thin green beans
10 broccolini
7 oz canned artichoke hearts (about 10 pieces)
generous pinch of saffron
2 tbsp olive oil
1 tbsp paprika
½ tsp ground turmeric
4 cups good-quality vegetable stock
1½ cups paella rice
1–2 lemons
salt and black pepper

Broiler on high, or grill pan on the highest heat | Baking sheet | Large frying or paella pan | Pestle and mortar (or use a mug and teaspoon) | Boiling water | Clean kitchen towels

Cut the bell pepper in half and cut out the stem and seeds | Lay the pieces on the baking sheet under a hot broiler, skin side up (or on a hot grill pan, skin side down) and heat until the skin blackens | Transfer to a plastic bag and seal inside | Leave to cool, then remove the skin | Cut the flesh into ½-inch strips

Meanwhile, drain the butter beans | Peel and finely chop the onion and garlic | Finely chop the tomato | Trim the green beans and cut off the heads of the broccolini | Cut the beans and broccolini stems only into ⅓–¾-inch pieces | Quarter the artichoke hearts | Set all the chopped veggies aside for later

Put the saffron threads in the dry frying or paella pan and place it over medium heat | Let it warm for about 1 minute to dry the saffron, then transfer to a mortar | Add a generous pinch of salt and pound with the pestle to grind them together

Add 1 tablespoon of the oil to the pan along with the bell pepper | Cook for 10–15 minutes, turning occasionally, until the peppers are soft but not browned | Remove from the pan and set aside about 6 strips | Cut the rest into ⅓–¾-inch pieces

Add the onion to the pan along with the remaining tablespoon oil | Cook for 10–15 minutes, until the onion has softened and browned a little, stirring occasionally | Add the garlic and cook for 2 minutes longer | Add the tomato and cook for about 10 minutes more, stirring from time to time, until the tomato pieces turn mushy | Stir in the salty saffron threads, paprika, turmeric, and a generous pinch of black pepper | Add the stock to the pan, turn up the heat and bring to a boil, then reduce the heat to medium

Stir in the green beans, butter beans, artichoke, and red bell pepper pieces (reserving the strips) | Increase the heat to bring the pan back to a simmer, then lower to medium | Taste the paella liquid—it should have a good "stock" taste that's a little too salty, so add a little more salt to the pan if necessary

Sprinkle the rice evenly over the pan | Bring it back to a boil, then reduce the heat to a fast simmer (medium-high) | Continue to simmer for 5 minutes without stirring | If you are using a large pan on a smaller burner you may need to move the pan around on the burner occasionally so that the rice cooks evenly across the pan

Decorate the surface of the paella with the red pepper strips and broccolini florets | Continue to cook without stirring for 10 minutes | Turn the broccolini a few times so that it cooks through, and check that the rice is still evenly distributed—you might need to use a spoon to move the rice in the pan

After 10 minutes, test the rice by biting a few grains | They should be translucent but al dente | If the pan starts to dry out before the rice is cooked, add a scant ½ cup boiling water by drizzling it through a strainer over the surface of the mixture (don't just pour it in) | If there is a lot of liquid visible when the rice is nearly cooked, consider either spooning some off or turning up the heat (a little bit of burning at the bottom of the pan is not considered a bad thing—the Valencians call it "socarrat," and treasure it)

Once the rice is cooked enough, give it a last short burst of heat to get any remaining liquid really bubbling, then turn off the heat and cover the top of the pan with foil and a couple of clean kitchen towels | Leave it for 10–15 minutes—this improves the taste and texture and allows the rice to absorb any excess stock | Cut the lemons into wedges and serve alongside the paella

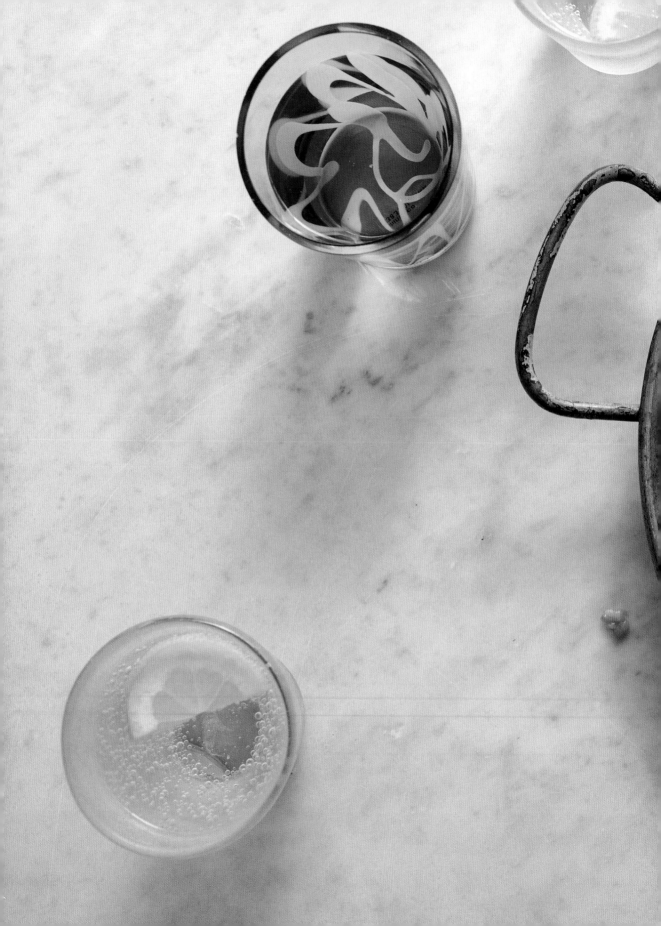

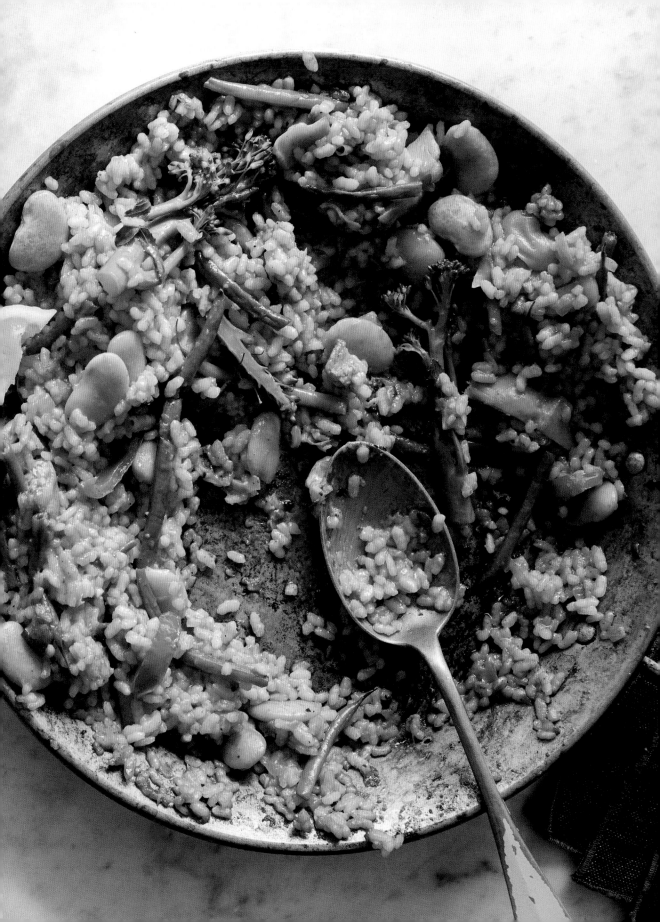

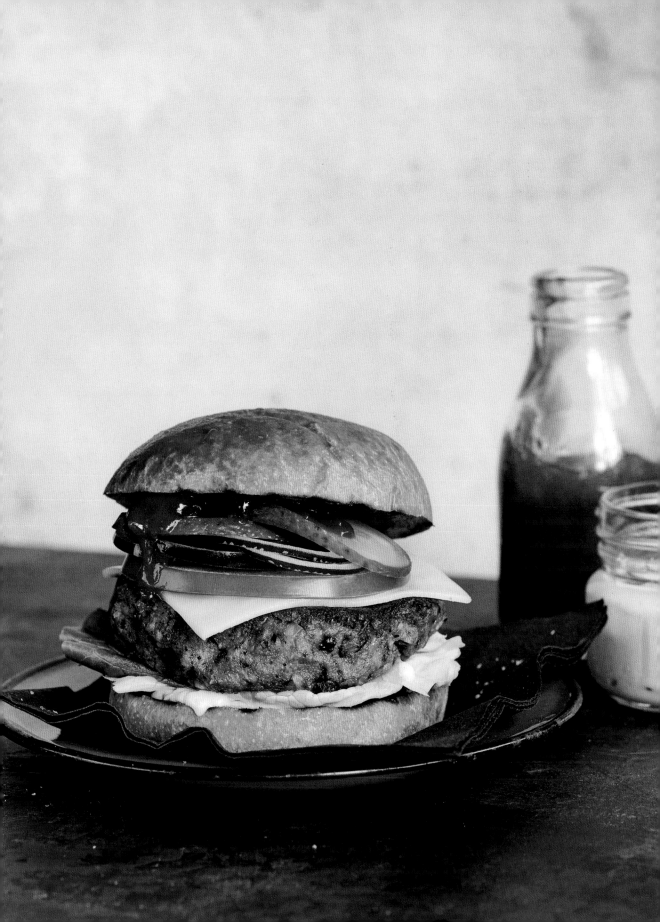

THE BIG BOSH! BURGER

We do love a good burger, and creating a big, meaty-tasting burger was high up on our list of priorities. This one gets its richness from sweet potatoes, black beans, and a whole host of spices. It's packed full of protein and the soft patty gives a good, filling bite. To make this even better, add a helping of Ultimate BBQ Coleslaw (page 148) to the top of the burger.

SERVES 6

14 oz sweet potatoes
1 onion
olive oil
1¼ cups cooked brown rice
3 tbsp breadcrumbs
½ tsp salt
½ tsp black pepper
½ tsp ground cumin
½ tsp garlic powder
½ tsp smoked paprika
2 tbsp all-purpose flour
1 can (15 oz) black beans

TO SERVE
1 beefsteak tomato
1 little gem lettuce
1 large red onion
6 burger buns
6 tsp ketchup
6 tsp vegan mayonnaise
12 slices dill pickle
6 slices dairy-free cheese

Preheat oven to 390°F | Line a baking sheet | Large frying pan over medium heat | Food processor

Peel the sweet potatoes and cut them into ¾-inch cubes | Put them on the lined baking sheet and bake for 30 minutes | Take them out of the oven and set aside

Meanwhile, peel and mince the onion | Pour a little oil into the frying pan | Put the onion in the pan and fry for 10–15 minutes, until very soft | Transfer the onion to a large bowl and wipe out the pan

Put the baked sweet potato in the food processor | Add the rice, breadcrumbs, salt, pepper, cumin, garlic powder, smoked paprika, and flour | Drain the black beans and add them to the food processor, then whizz everything up to a thick paste | Scrape the paste into the bowl with the onions and mix everything together with a spoon

Add a little oil to the pan and set it over medium-high heat | Divide the mixture into six and use your hands to mold them into patty shapes | Place the patties in the hot pan and fry for 3 minutes on each side, until golden

While the burgers are cooking, slice the tomato into 6 thin slices | Separate the leaves of the lettuce and peel and slice the onion into thin rings

Build your burgers by placing them inside the burger buns, topping with ketchup, vegan mayo, and slices of tomato and pickle, lettuce, red onion, and dairy-free cheese

RICH & CREAMY LASAGNA

This lasagna is easy enough to make and will impress your dinner guests no end. The béchamel is creamy as hell and as long as there are no overlaps, the pasta will cook to perfection. This is perfect dinner-party fodder, or a treat for you and your loved one that will leave lots of leftovers—it may be even better the next day. Check out the photo on page 122.

SERVES 8

1 butternut squash (about 2¼ lb)
3 medium eggplants (about 1 lb 10 oz)
1 tsp chili powder
¼ cup olive oil, plus extra for greasing
3 tbsp balsamic vinegar
21 oz baby spinach
1 lb dried lasagna sheets
a few sprigs fresh rosemary, to serve

FOR THE TOMATO SAUCE

1 oz dried porcini mushrooms
¼ cup olive oil
1 red onion
5 garlic cloves
1 carrot
2 celery stalks
1 red bell pepper
3 sprigs fresh rosemary
⅔ cup red wine
2 cans (14.5 oz each) chopped tomatoes
1 tsp superfine sugar
salt and black pepper

FOR THE BÉCHAMEL

3½ oz cashews
1 garlic clove
¾ cup + 2 tbsp unsweetened plant-
    based milk
3½ tbsp dairy-free butter or spread
3 tbsp all-purpose flour
5 tbsp nutritional yeast, optional
2 tsp onion powder
½ lemon
7 tbsp water
salt and black pepper

Preheat oven to 350°F | Line 2 large baking sheets | Brush the inside of a 9 x 13-inch lasagna dish with oil | Boiling water | Large deep frying pan or Dutch oven over medium heat | Food processor, optional | Large saucepan with lid | Small saucepan | Medium saucepan | Blender

Put the porcini mushrooms for the tomato sauce into a large mug and cover with boiling water, then set aside

Peel the squash, cut it in half, and scoop out and discard the seeds | Trim the eggplants and cut the squash and eggplant into ⅓-inch slices | Put them in a bowl with the chili powder and 3 tablespoons of the olive oil and toss to coat | Lay the squash on one lined baking sheet, the eggplant on the other | Put both pans in the oven and roast for 45 minutes

Meanwhile, make the tomato sauce | Heat the olive oil in the large deep frying pan or Dutch oven | Peel and finely dice the onion and add it to the pan to soften for 3 minutes | Peel and mince the garlic, add to the pan, and cook for 3 minutes longer

Trim and roughly chop the carrot and celery | Cut the bell pepper in half and cut out the stem and seeds | Remove the leaves from the rosemary sprigs by running your thumb and forefinger from the top to the base of the stems (the leaves should easily come away) | Put the carrot, celery, bell pepper, and rosemary leaves in the food processor and pulse a few times until all the veg are finely chopped (or do this by hand)

Add the chopped veg to the pan with the onion and garlic | Stir and cook for 15 minutes | Pour in the red wine, increase the heat to medium-high, and cook for 5–7 minutes, until the wine has cooked off but left everything a lovely red color

Scoop the porcini out of the mug and finely chop | Add to the pan with the liquid from the mug, the chopped tomatoes, and the sugar | Stir and simmer for 10 minutes longer

Remove the pans from the oven | Drizzle the eggplant with the balsamic vinegar and mix well | If the butternut squash is very wet, drain it in a sieve, pressing out the liquid | Transfer to a large bowl and quickly mash

Add the eggplant to the tomato sauce and simmer for 20 minutes, stirring occasionally, until the sauce has thickened | Taste and season with salt and pepper | Take off the heat and set aside

Put the remaining 1 tablespoon oil into the large saucepan and place it over medium heat | Add the spinach and cover with a lid | Cook for about 5 minutes until wilted | Transfer to a sieve and squeeze out as much liquid as you can (or place in a clean kitchen towel and wring it out)

Now make the béchamel | Set a small saucepan of water over high heat and bring to a boil | Add the cashews and boil for 10 minutes | Peel and mince the garlic

Set a medium saucepan over medium heat | Warm the plant-based milk in the microwave | Put the dairy-free butter in the pan and stir with a wooden spoon until it melts, then turn the heat right down and gradually add the flour, stirring vigorously until you have a doughy paste | Gradually pour in the warm plant-based milk, stirring all the time until you have a thick, creamy sauce | Keep stirring until the sauce thickens to the consistency of custard | Add the garlic, nutritional yeast, if using, onion powder, plus a pinch of salt and pepper | Squeeze in the lemon juice, catching any seeds with your other hand | Stir to mix together

Drain the cashews and rinse with cold water | Put them into the blender with the 7 tbsp water | Blend to a fine cream with no bits | Pour the béchamel into the blender and blend everything together

Cover the bottom of the greased lasagna dish with lasagna sheets, breaking them if necessary to make a complete and unbroken layer that will seal in the steam and properly cook the pasta | Spoon a third of the tomato sauce over the bottom of the lasagna | Lay a third of the spinach on top, followed by a third of the squash | Drizzle over a quarter of the béchamel sauce | Repeat twice more with layers of pasta, then tomato sauce, spinach, squash, and béchamel | Top with a final layer of pasta, using broken pieces to fill any gaps (try to avoid overlaps), and cover with the remaining béchamel | Put a few rosemary leaves on top to garnish

Cover the lasagna with foil and put in the oven on the lowest rack | Bake for 50 minutes | Remove the foil and bake for 15 minutes longer; stand for 10 minutes | Serve with a green salad and a little balsamic glaze

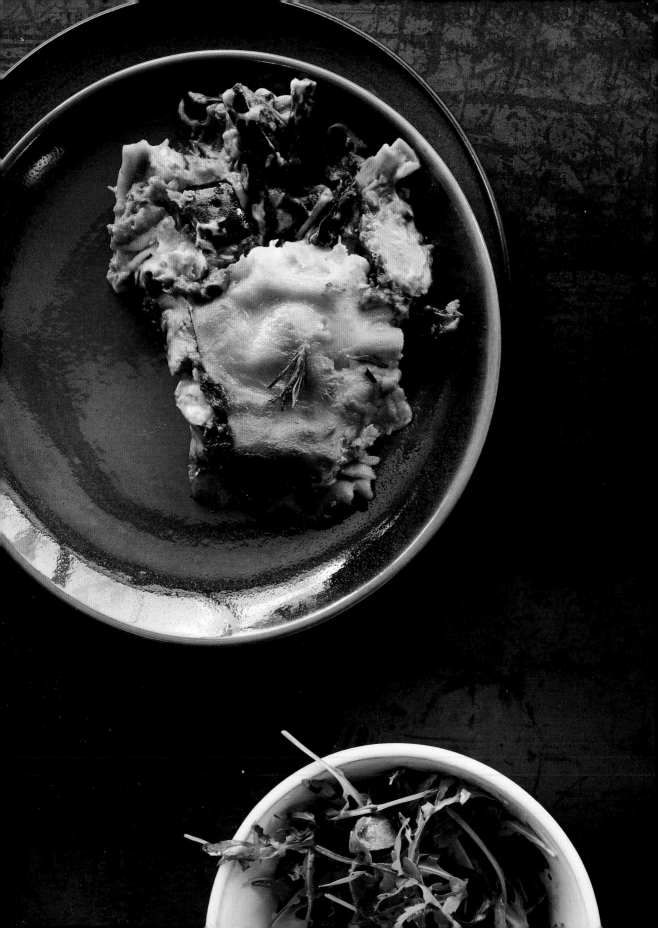

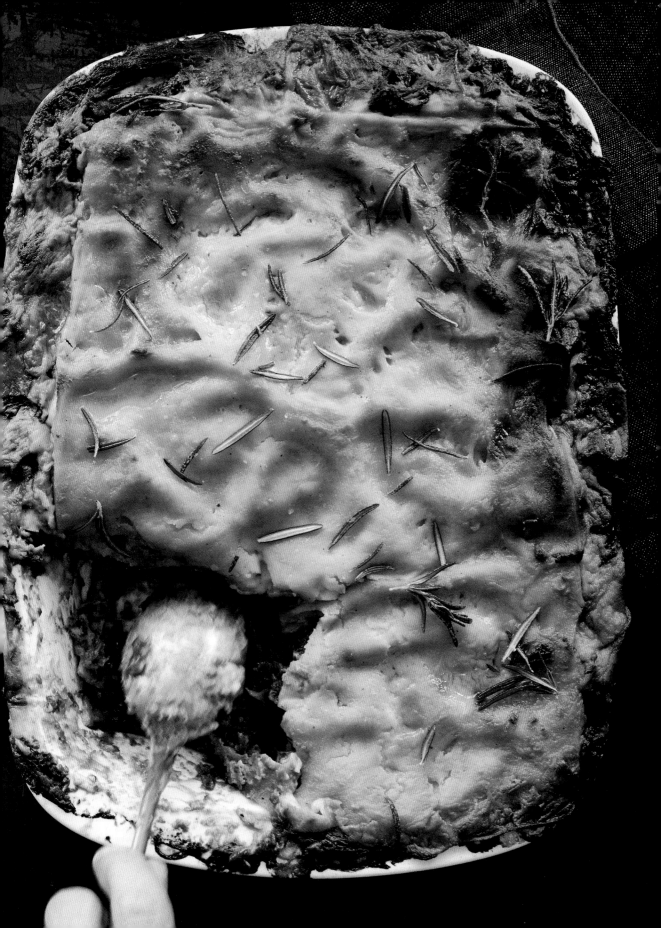

SPIRAL TART

This dish will test your arrangement skills (plus your patience!), but it's worth it for the photo-worthy result. This healthy tart is full of freshly roasted veggies with an ever-so-slightly spicy tomato base. It's best to use a peeler to get the optimum thickness, and make sure the height of the veggie strips is consistent for a nice, even tart.

SERVES 4–6

11 oz refrigerated pie dough
flour, for dusting
5 tbsp tomato puree
½–1 tsp chili flakes
1 oz fresh basil
1 tbsp balsamic glaze
3 eggplants
4 large carrots
3 zucchini
2 tbsp olive oil
salt and black pepper

Preheat oven to 350°F | Clean work surface dusted liberally with flour | Rolling pin (or use a clean, dry wine bottle) | Large bowl filled with water | 8–8½-inch tart pan with a removable bottom

Unravel the pie dough and roll it out on the floured work surface until it's a scant ¼ inch thick | Drape it over the rolling pin and lift it into the tart pan | Gently press the pastry into the edges of the pan with your fingers to line the bottom and sides | Use a knife to cut off the excess at the top of the pan

Spoon the tomato puree onto the bottom and spread it out evenly with the back of the spoon | Sprinkle with the chili flakes | Pick the basil leaves from the bunch and arrange them in an even layer all over the bottom | Drizzle with the balsamic glaze and set aside

Trim the ends from the eggplants, carrots, and zucchini and slice the eggplant in half lengthwise | Use a vegetable peeler to slice each into thin ribbons and put them into the bowl filled with water to soak for about 3 minutes (this makes them more supple and easier to shape) | Remove and pat dry with paper towels

Take 1 ribbon of each of the vegetables and lay them on top of one another, first zucchini, then carrot, then eggplant | Roll them up into a tight spiral to resemble a rose | Place the spiral in the middle of the tart | Start spiraling the ribbons tightly from the central rose all the way out to the edges, alternating from zucchini, to carrot, to eggplant

Once the tart is completely full of vegetables, season with salt and pepper and drizzle with the oil | Put the pan in the preheated oven and bake for 40 minutes | Test and if you prefer softer vegetables, cover with foil and bake 15–20 minutes longer | Take the pan out of the oven and slide the tart out of the pan

Bring your work of art to the table so that everyone can take a photo, then carefully cut into slices with a VERY sharp knife

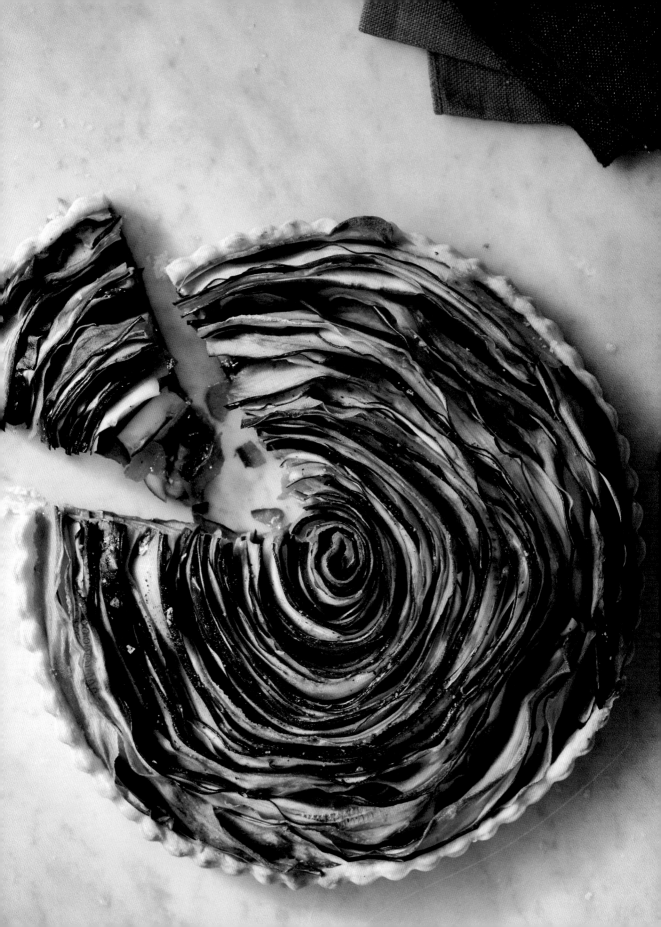

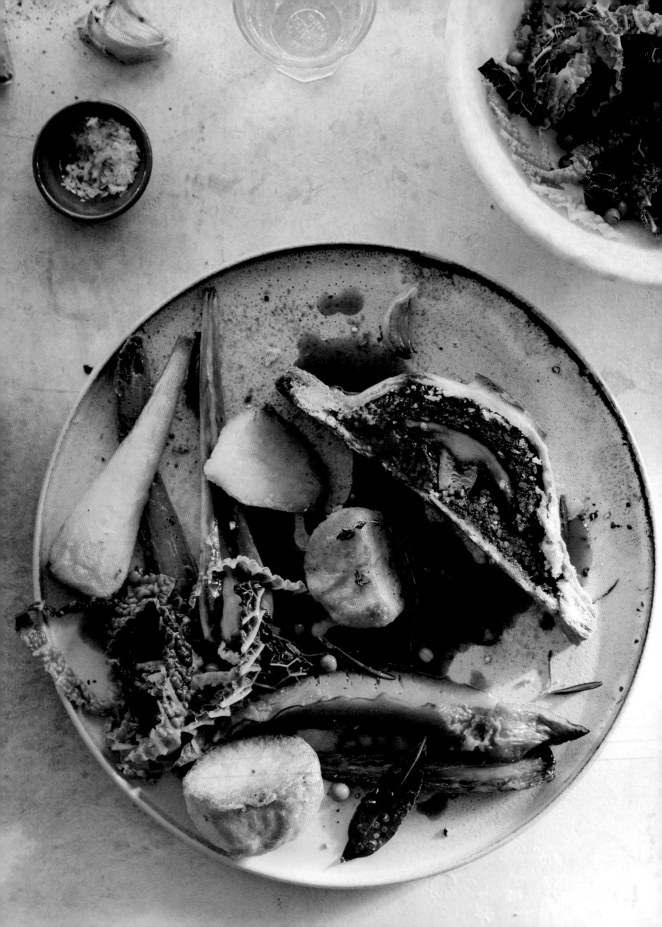

THE BIG BOSH! ROAST

Whether it's Christmas, Thanksgiving, or just a normal Sunday, a roast dinner is the epitome of traditional food. We've based ours around a glorious centerpiece mushroom Wellington, one that is rich, full of texture, and incredibly moreish, and goes great with any gravy. This meal should satisfy even the fussiest of dinner guests.

SERVES 4–6 WITH LEFTOVERS

Rosemary & Thyme Roast Vegetables ingredients (see page 130)
Mushroom Wellington ingredients (see page 128)
Red Wine Gravy ingredients (see page 131)

Preheat oven to 390°F | Line 2 baking sheets with parchment paper | 1 large empty saucepan with a lid | 1 large saucepan of boiling water over high heat | Large deep roasting pan | Shallow sheet pan | Large deep frying pan | Food processor | Pastry brush, optional | Pastry cutters, optional

Start with the Rosemary & Thyme Roast Vegetables by peeling and boiling the potatoes and parsnips following the instructions on page 130, up to the point when they're on their baking sheets and cooling to room temperature

Meanwhile, assemble the Mushroom Wellington following the instructions on page 128 | Once the Wellington is ready to go in the oven, set it aside while you get on with the roast vegetables

Finish preparing the roast vegetables and put the baking sheet on the second rack of the oven, leaving enough space for the Wellington to fit on the top rack later | Set the timer for 20 minutes

Start preparing the vegetables for the Red Wine Gravy following the instructions on page 131

When the timer goes off, put the Wellington on the top rack of the oven and take out the roast vegetables | Gently shake the pan and return it to the oven | Set a timer for 30 minutes

15 minutes before the timer goes off, finish making the Red Wine Gravy | Take the roast vegetables and Wellington out of the oven and transfer to serving dishes | Serve!

MUSHROOM WELLINGTON

SERVES 6

7 garlic cloves

5 sprigs fresh rosemary

6 sprigs fresh thyme

4 small portobello mushrooms (about 10.5 oz)

1 tsp + 1 tbsp olive oil

1 tsp salt, plus a little extra

2 tsp black pepper, plus a little extra

1 large red onion

2 tsp light brown sugar

10 oz cremini mushrooms

½ cup white wine

7 oz vacuum-packed chestnuts

9 oz pecans

2 slices seeded bread (about 3 oz)

2 sheets refrigerated rectangular vegan pie dough (16 × 10-inch)

¼ cup unsweetened plant-based milk

Preheat oven to 390°F | Line 2 baking sheets with parchment paper | Large frying pan over medium heat | Food processor | Pastry brush, optional | Pastry cutters, optional

Peel and mince 4 of the garlic cloves using a sharp knife | Remove the leaves from 4 rosemary and 4 thyme sprigs by running your thumb and forefinger from the top to the base of the stems (the leaves should easily come away), then finely chop

Lay the portobello mushrooms on one of the lined baking sheets with the stems pointing up | Drizzle 1 teaspoon oil over the gills of each mushroom and sprinkle with a little salt and pepper | Divide the chopped rosemary, thyme, and garlic among the mushrooms | Put the pan in the oven and cook for 15 minutes | Remove and set aside

Meanwhile, peel and finely chop the red onion | Add the tablespoon of oil to the frying pan | Add the red onion to the pan and sauté for 10 minutes, stirring regularly, until softened

While the onions are cooking, peel and finely chop the remaining 3 garlic cloves | Remove the leaves from the remaining rosemary and thyme sprigs and finely chop | Measure 1 teaspoon salt, 1 teaspoon of the pepper, and the sugar into a small bowl | Add the garlic, rosemary, thyme, salt, pepper, and sugar into the pan and stir everything around for 1 minute

Put the cremini mushrooms into the food processor and whizz until very finely chopped | Tip them into the pan, increase the heat to high, and cook until softened and all the liquid has evaporated, about 5–7 minutes

Pour the white wine into the pan and stir it around for about 3 minutes, or until almost all the liquid has cooked off | Tip the mixture into a large mixing bowl and leave to cool for 5 minutes

Put the chestnuts, pecans, and bread into the food processor and whizz until they resemble breadcrumbs (you may need to do this in batches) | Add to the bowl with the onions | Using a wooden spoon, thoroughly stir everything together until you have a thick dough-like mixture

Lay 1 sheet of pie dough on the other lined baking sheet | Spread half the chestnut mixture lengthwise down the middle of the pastry sheet | Use your hands to mold the chestnut mixture into a rectangle shape with a flat top, leaving at least a 1¼-inch gap on all four sides | This shape will dictate the shape of the Wellington, so make sure it's nice and straight and level on top

Place the 4 cooked portobello mushrooms neatly on top of the chestnut mixture, stems facing up, making sure the sides of the mushrooms don't hang off the edges | Layer the rest of the chestnut mixture over the top, encasing the mushrooms | Smooth and shape into a neat, long, rectangular mound

Using a pastry brush or your finger, brush a little of the plant-based milk around the exposed pastry edge | Lay the second pastry sheet over the mushroom filling and press it all down well, ensuring there are no air bubbles | Seal the edges by pushing down all the way around the filling with your fingers | Trim any excess pastry from the edges, making sure you leave a ½-inch raised border around the base of the Wellington | Set the excess pastry aside for later | Use a fork to crimp all around the edges of the pastry to firmly seal the Wellington and to make it look nice

Roll out the excess pastry if necessary and use a pastry cutter to cut out shapes | Brush the Wellington lightly with the plant-based milk and decorate the top with the pastry shapes | Brush the shapes with the plant-based milk | Pierce some air vents in the top of the Wellington with a fork or sharp knife

Put the Wellington in the oven and bake it for 40 minutes, checking after 30 minutes (if it looks ready, remove it from the oven) | Use a bread knife to carefully cut the Wellington into slices and serve

ROSEMARY & THYME ROAST VEGETABLES

SERVES 4–6

2¾ lb russet or other fluffy potatoes
5 medium carrots
5 medium parsnips
1 small butternut squash
   (about 1 lb 5 oz)
1 garlic bulb + 5 cloves
1 tbsp salt, plus a little extra
½ cup olive oil
16 sprigs fresh thyme
8 sprigs fresh rosemary

Preheat oven to 390°F | 1 large empty saucepan with a lid | 1 large saucepan of boiling water over high heat | Large deep roasting pan | Shallow sheet pan

Peel the potatoes, carrots, parsnips, and butternut squash

Cut the carrots and parsnips lengthwise into halves or quarters and cut out any tough cores from the parsnips | Seed the butternut squash, then cut it into roughly the same size pieces as the carrots | Break the garlic bulb into cloves and lightly squash them with the side of the knife

Cut the potatoes into thirds or quarters and put them in one of the saucepans | Fill the pan with cold water, sprinkle in the tablespoon of salt (to make them extra fluffy), and set the pan over high heat | Bring to a boil and then cook for 5–8 minutes

Meanwhile, put the parsnips into the other pan and boil for 5 minutes | Drain and transfer to the large, deep roasting pan to cool down

Put the butternut squash and carrots into the sheet pan and toss in 3 tablespoons of the oil, half the thyme sprigs, and half the rosemary | Sprinkle with salt to taste | Toss it all together and set aside

When they're done, drain the potatoes and tip them back into the pan | Put the lid on and shake the pan for 15 seconds to scuff the outsides of the potatoes, then tip them into the roasting pan next to the parsnips and let them cool down to room temperature

Nestle the remaining thyme and rosemary sprigs and the garlic cloves you squashed earlier in among the potatoes and parsnips | Pour the remaining olive oil over them and toss gently to coat

Put the pan with the potatoes on the second rack of the hot oven and the pan with the carrots underneath (leave enough space above the top rack for the Wellington if you're making the full roast) and cook for 50–60 minutes | Toss the veg every 20 minutes to ensure they are evenly cooked on all sides | They should be golden and crispy on the outside when they're done | If you want to give them an extra crispy boost at the end, turn on the broiler and place one pan at a time under it | Keep a close eye on it; they should crisp up within just a few minutes

RED WINE GRAVY

A good gravy is the jewel in the crown of a great roast dinner, and this is a really good gravy. Try it drizzled over a plate of hot French fries for an indulgent Yorkshire classic.

SERVES 6

Deep frying pan with a lid over medium heat

1 red onion
1 small carrot
1 celery stalk
2 tbsp olive oil
3 garlic cloves
1 sprig fresh rosemary
2 sprigs fresh thyme
1½ cups red wine
4 cups vegetable stock
3 tbsp cornstarch
6 tbsp room-temperature water
1 tbsp tomato paste
1 tsp yeast extract (e.g., Marmite)
1 tsp English mustard, prepared
1 tsp dark brown sugar
½ tsp salt
½ tsp black pepper

Peel and finely dice the red onion, carrot, and celery, keeping them separate on the cutting board

Pour the olive oil into the hot pan | Add the diced onion and cook for 2 minutes | Peel and crush the garlic cloves into the pan and stir everything together | Cook for 2 minutes until you've released the aroma of the garlic

Add the diced carrot and celery and the rosemary and thyme sprigs | Stir everything together on the heat for about 7 minutes, until the vegetables are well softened | Pour in the red wine and cook until most of the liquid has evaporated

Pour the vegetable stock into the pan | Turn up the heat so that it's bubbling nicely, then reduce to a gentle simmer, put the lid on, and cook for 10 minutes

Take the pan off the heat and strain the liquid into a bowl through a sieve so that you're left with a clear stock | Pour it back into the pan and put it back on the heat

Put the cornstarch into a small glass | Add the water and mix together with a fork, stirring really well to ensure there are no lumps

Add the cornstarch mixture to the pan and whisk continuously while the gravy bubbles away for 5 minutes, until you have a nice, thick consistency | Add the tomato paste, yeast extract, mustard, sugar, salt, and pepper and stir until well mixed | Pour the gravy into a pitcher ready to serve

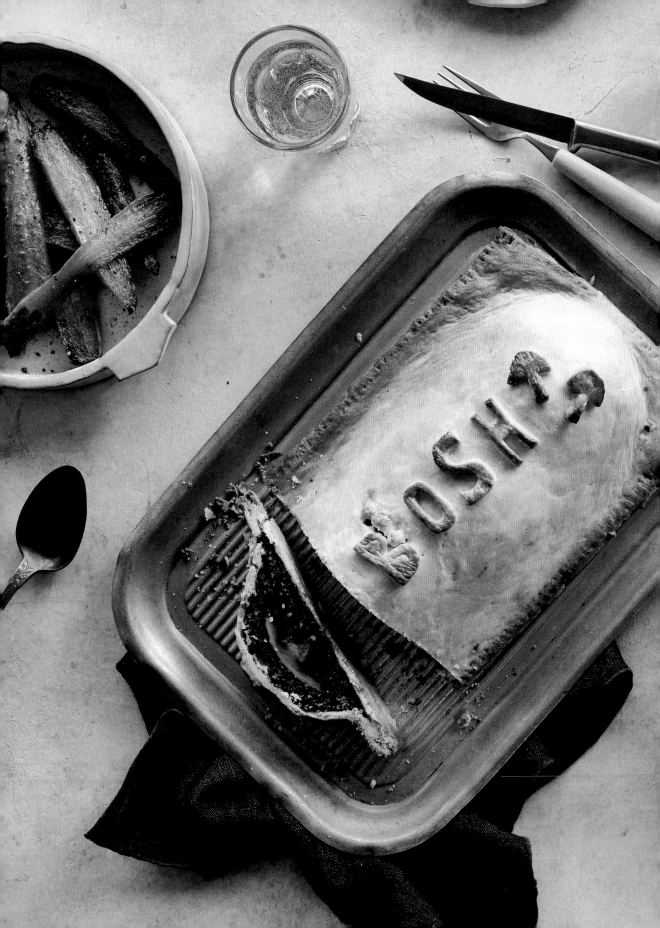

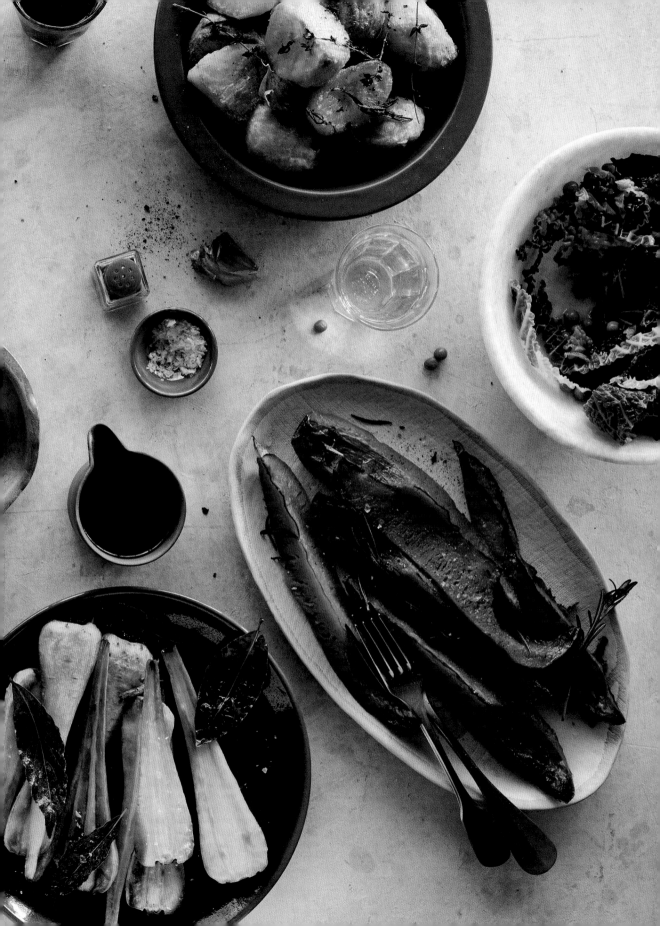

"FISH" & CHIPS

Reminiscent of a trip to the seaside, this dish is a great nod to the pub classic. A crunchy outer and soft middle give the tofu goujons a satisfying bite and the lemon and tartare sauce add a wonderful sharpness. Add some luxurious chunky fries and you have a dish to die for—check out page 137 if you don't believe us! Pass the salt and vinegar.

SERVES 4

2 containers (10 oz each) extra-firm tofu
Tartare Sauce ingredients (see page 136)
4 large russet or other fluffy potatoes
    (about 1kg)
3 sheets nori
Minted Mushy Peas ingredients (see
    page 136)
vegetable oil, for deep-frying
ketchup, to serve
2 lemons, to serve
sea salt

FOR THE MARINADE
1 lemon
generous ¾ cup white wine
1 tbsp caper brine
    (from a jar of capers)
1 tsp salt

FOR THE BATTER
1⅓ cups all-purpose flour
5 tbsp cornstarch
½ tsp salt
½ tsp black pepper
1 cup ale

Tofu press or use 2 clean kitchen towels and a weight such as a heavy book | Large saucepan | Clean kitchen towel | Scissors | Toothpicks | Small saucepan | Large deep saucepan | Thermometer, optional | Cover 2 large plates with paper towels | 2 baking sheets

Press the tofu using a tofu press or place it between two clean kitchen towels, lay it on a plate, and put a weight on top | Leave for at least 30 minutes to drain any liquid and firm up before you start cooking

Once the tofu is pressed, drain away any liquid that has collected on the plate | Cut the block lengthwise down the middle so that you have 2 long rectangles, then cut across each rectangle to make 8 even-sized blocks | You should end up with 16 tofu pieces that are all the same size

Make the marinade by cutting the lemon in half and squeezing the juice over a bowl, catching any seeds with your other hand | Add the white wine, caper brine, and salt and stir to combine | Add the tofu, turning to cover it in the marinade | Set aside to marinate, turning the tofu occasionally

Make the Tartare Sauce following the instructions on page 136 and set aside

Fill the large saucepan with water and bring it to a boil over high heat | Peel the potatoes and cut them into ⅓-inch-thick French fry shapes | Tip them into the hot water, bring it back to a boil, and cook for 5 minutes | Drain the potatoes, spread them out over a clean kitchen towel, and leave them to dry

To make the batter, put the flour, cornstarch, salt, and pepper into a mixing bowl and stir to mix | Slowly pour in the ale, whisking continuously so that no lumps form | Set aside once you have a smooth batter

Use scissors to cut 16 rectangles of nori the same size as the sides of the tofu blocks | Take a piece of tofu out of the marinade and stick one of the nori pieces to it (the wetness of the tofu will help it stick) | Hold the nori in place with 2 toothpicks | Repeat so that all the tofu pieces have a piece of nori on one side

Make the Minted Mushy Peas following the recipe on page 136 and set aside

Heat the oven to 350°F | Cut the 2 lemons into wedges for serving

Pour the vegetable oil into the deep saucepan so that it comes no more than two-thirds up the side of the pan | Set the pan over medium-high and heat to about 285°F (this is a fairly low temperature for deep-frying so if you don't have a thermometer, put a piece of potato in the pan to test the temperature: when it's ready the potato should float but take a little while to brown)

Put half the fries in the hot oil and deep-fry for 3–4 minutes, then take them out with a slotted spoon and spread them out on the paper towels for a few minutes to cool down slightly | Put the rest of the potatoes into the oil and repeat, spreading them over the other plate of paper towels to cool | Turn up the heat and get the oil really hot, around 355°F (this should make a wooden spoon dipped in the oil sizzle around the edges)

Carefully put the first batch of fries back in the hot oil and fry them for 4–5 minutes, until they're really golden and crispy | Take the fries out of the oil with a slotted spoon and spread them over one of the baking sheets | Sprinkle the fries with sea salt and put the pan in the oven to keep the fries warm | Bring the oil back up to 355°F and tip in the second batch of fries | After 4–5 minutes, remove and spread over the second baking sheet

Get the oil back up to 355°F and line the plates with fresh paper towels

Take the nori-lined tofu blocks and dip them into the batter in batches, turning them carefully so that they're completely covered | Carefully drop the battered tofu "fish" into the hot oil and fry for 3–4 minutes, until they're dark golden brown all over (you may need to cook them in batches if there isn't much room and so that the temperature of the oil doesn't drop too low) | Remove the tofu "fish" with a slotted spoon and drain the pieces on paper towels for 30 seconds, then carefully remove the toothpicks | Repeat so that all the tofu blocks are double-dipped in two coats of batter

Take the fries out of the oven and immediately serve on warm plates | Divide the crispy tofu "fish" pieces among the plates and add large spoonfuls of Minted Mushy Peas and Tartare Sauce | Serve with tomato ketchup and the lemon wedges to squeeze over the tofu "fish" pieces

MINTED MUSHY PEAS

SERVES 4

1 package (10 oz) frozen peas
1 tbsp dairy-free butter or spread
10 fresh mint leaves
½ lemon
½ tsp salt
½ tsp black pepper

Small saucepan of boiling water over high heat

Pour the peas into the boiling water and bring back to a boil | Cook for 3 minutes | While the peas are cooking, put the rest of the ingredients into a bowl and mix together with a fork | Drain the peas and add them to the other ingredients | Blend lightly with a stick blender while the peas are still hot, ensuring roughly half of them remain whole | Stir to mix in all the seasoning

TARTARE SAUCE

SERVES 4

1 small shallot
½ lemon
½ tsp + a pinch of salt
1½ tbsp capers
4 tsp minced cornichons
1½ tbsp chopped fresh tarragon
2 tbsp chopped fresh chives
1 tbsp chopped fresh parsley
scant ½ cup vegan mayonnaise

Peel and finely slice the shallot and put it into a bowl | Squeeze in the juice of the half lemon, catching any seeds in your other hand, and add the pinch of salt | Add the capers, cornichons, tarragon, chives, and parsley to the bowl | Add the vegan mayo and the ½ teaspoon of salt, and stir everything together

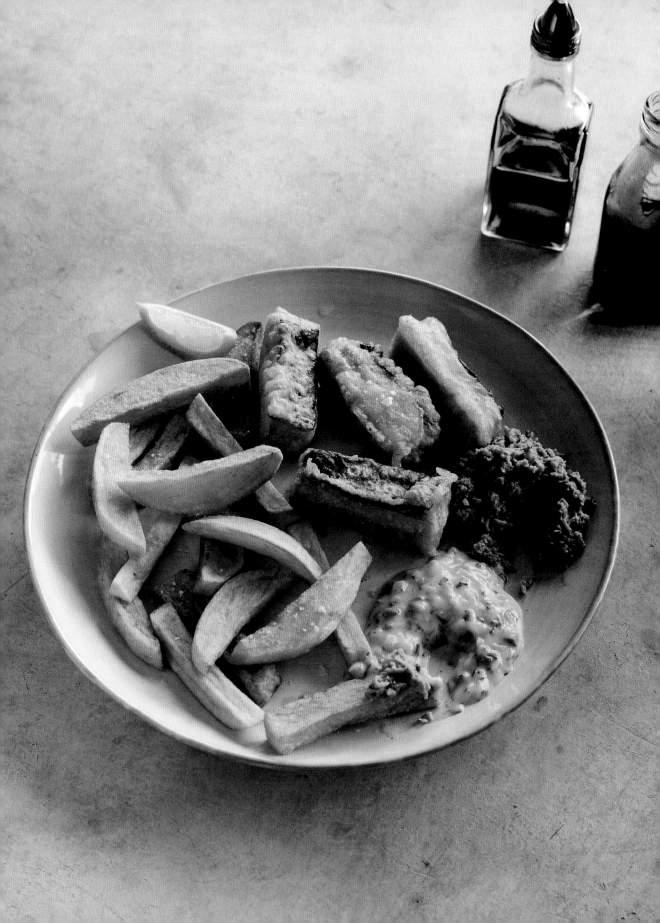

WORLD'S BEST PESTO LASAGNA

We've been cooking and refining this pesto lasagna dish for years. It's an absolute showstopper: rich, flavorful, and healthy(ish). It'll take you a while to make since there are a few different parts to combine, but it's so worth it—see the photos overleaf. Use light olive oil for a light, delicious pesto.

SERVES 8

2 eggplants
2 zucchini
2 yellow bell peppers
2 red bell peppers
1 tbsp olive oil
12 lasagna sheets
salt and black pepper

FOR THE TOMATO SAUCE

2 tbsp olive oil
1 red onion
3 garlic cloves
3½ oz pitted black olives
4 tbsp capers
3 cups tomato puree

FOR THE BÉCHAMEL

5 oz cashews
scant 2 cups unsweetened plant-based milk
3½ tbsp dairy-free butter or spread
3 tbsp all-purpose flour
5 tbsp nutritional yeast
2 tsp onion powder
1 garlic clove
½ lemon
7 tbsp water

FOR THE PESTO

2½ oz pine nuts
2 oz fresh basil leaves
3 tbsp nutritional yeast
2 garlic cloves
½ lemon
⅔ cup light olive oil

Preheat oven to 350°F | 3 baking sheets | Large saucepan over medium heat | Small saucepan over high heat | Medium saucepan over medium heat | Blender | 12 x 8-inch baking dish

Trim the eggplants and zucchini and cut them diagonally into slices about ⅓ inch thick | Cut the bell peppers in half and cut out the stems and seeds, then cut them in half again | Divide the chopped vegetables between two of the baking sheets, drizzle with the oil, and sprinkle with a good pinch of salt and pepper | Put the pans in the hot oven and roast for 20 minutes, then remove and set aside

Next, make the tomato sauce | Pour the oil into the large saucepan | Peel and finely chop the onion and add it to the pan | Cook for 5–10 minutes, until soft | Peel and crush the garlic cloves into the pan, cooking for 2 minutes | Drain and roughly chop the olives and add them to the pan along with the capers, tomato puree, and a good pinch of salt and pepper | Reduce the heat to medium-low and leave to simmer for 25–30 minutes, stirring occasionally

Meanwhile, put the cashews in the small saucepan, cover with water, and bring to a boil | Boil for 10 minutes

To make the béchamel sauce, warm the plant-based milk in the microwave | Put the dairy-free butter in the medium saucepan and stir with a wooden spoon until it melts, then turn the heat right down and gradually add the flour to the pan, stirring vigorously until you have a doughy paste | Gradually pour in the warm plant-based milk, stirring all the time until you have a thick, creamy sauce | Keep stirring until the sauce thickens to the consistency of custard | Add the nutritional yeast and the onion powder | Peel and crush the garlic clove and add it to the pan | Squeeze the lemon juice into the pan, catching any seeds with your other hand

Drain the boiled cashews and rinse them with cold water to cool them down | Put them in the blender along with the water | Whizz to a fine cream with no bits | Pour the béchamel sauce into the blender and whizz together | Season with salt and pepper | Pour into a bowl and set aside | Clean out the blender

To make the pesto, spread the pine nuts over the clean baking sheet, put it in the oven, and toast for 3 minutes | Put them in the blender along with the basil and the nutritional yeast | Peel the garlic cloves and add them to the blender | Squeeze in the lemon juice, catching any seeds with your other hand | Pour in the olive oil | Blitz everything together until you've made a fine pesto | Taste and season with salt and pepper

Cover the bottom and sides of the baking dish with a thin layer of tomato sauce | Put a layer of lasagna sheets over the bottom, without overlapping them | Use broken up bits of lasagna to cover any gaps or corners

Spread a third of the remaining tomato sauce onto the lasagna sheets | Place a third of the baked veggies on top | Spread a third of the cashew béchamel on top, spreading it all the way to the edges of the dish | Drizzle a third of the pesto sauce on top | Repeat twice more, making layers of pasta, tomato sauce, veggies, and cashew sauce and topping with a long, arty drizzle of pesto

Cover the dish with foil, put it in the oven, and bake for 45 minutes | Remove the foil and bake for 10 more minutes | Take it out of the oven and leave it to stand for 10 minutes before serving

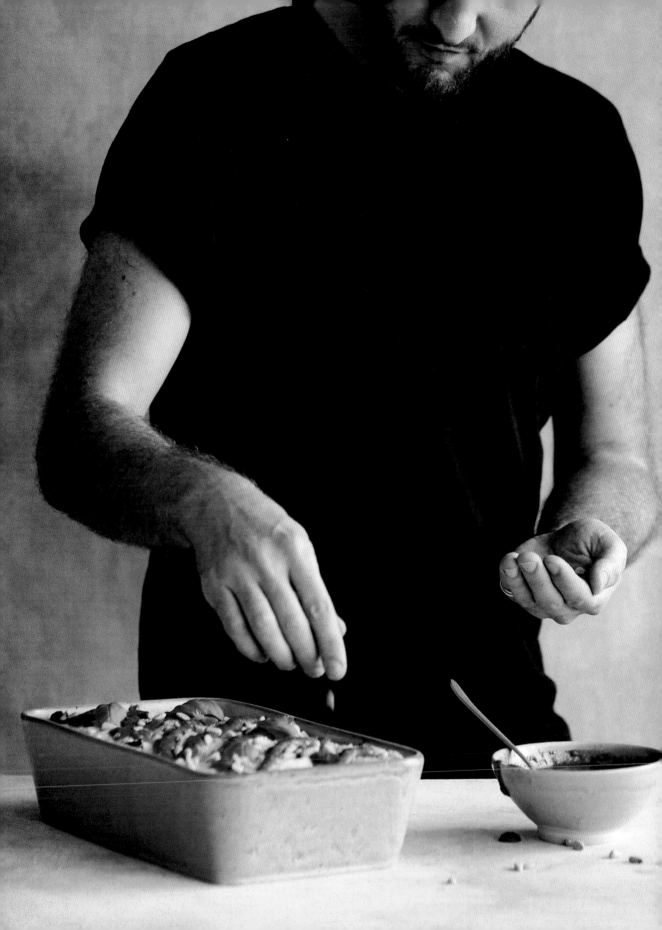

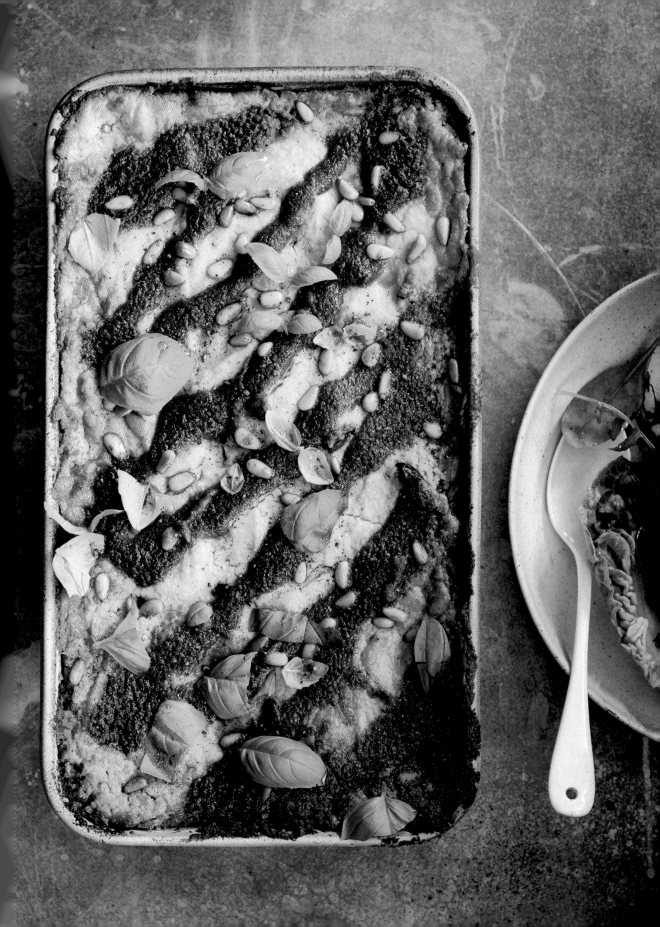

04

GREENS
& BOSH!
BOWLS

It's protein o'clock
Get real healthy with BOSH! Bowls
And amazing greens

TOMATO & POMEGRANATE SALAD

This dish is extremely colorful and tasty. The zingy fresh tomato contrasts with the sweet, juicy bursts of the pomegranate seeds and the explosion of flavor from the fresh herbs. This surprising flavor combination creates the perfect sharing side salad for an Italian pasta, or would serve as a super-healthy light meal or side for a BBQ.

SERVES 4–6

2 slices whole wheat bread
¼ cup olive oil
1 lemon
1 tsp brown sugar
4 drops Tabasco, optional
14 oz baby tomatoes
1 small red onion
handful fresh parsley
handful fresh mint
1 pomegranate or
   3½ oz pomegranate seeds
⅔ cup pea shoots or other salad greens
salt and black pepper

Medium frying pan over low heat

Cut the bread into ⅓-inch cubes | Heat 1 tablespoon of the olive oil in the pan and sauté the bread cubes for 2–3 minutes, tossing regularly until they are browned on all sides | Tip onto a plate and set aside

Cut the lemon in half and squeeze the juice into a large bowl, catching any seeds in your other hand | Stir in the remaining 3 tablespoons of oil and the brown sugar and season with the salt and pepper and Tabasco, if using | Taste and adjust the seasoning if necessary

Halve the tomatoes, peel and finely slice the red onion, pick the leaves from the parsley and mint, and add them all to the bowl | Remove the seeds from the pomegranate by rolling it first to loosen the seeds, then scoring around the middle and prising the two halves apart | Hold the halves over the bowl and tap the bottom of each half firmly with a spoon to release the seeds | Add the salad greens and croutons, toss gently, and serve to impressed guests

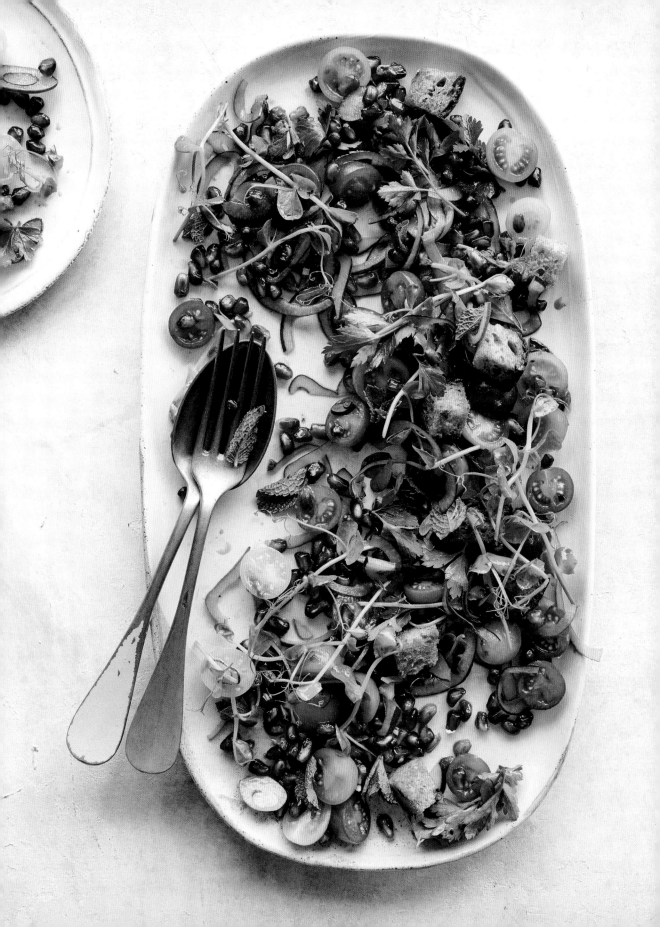

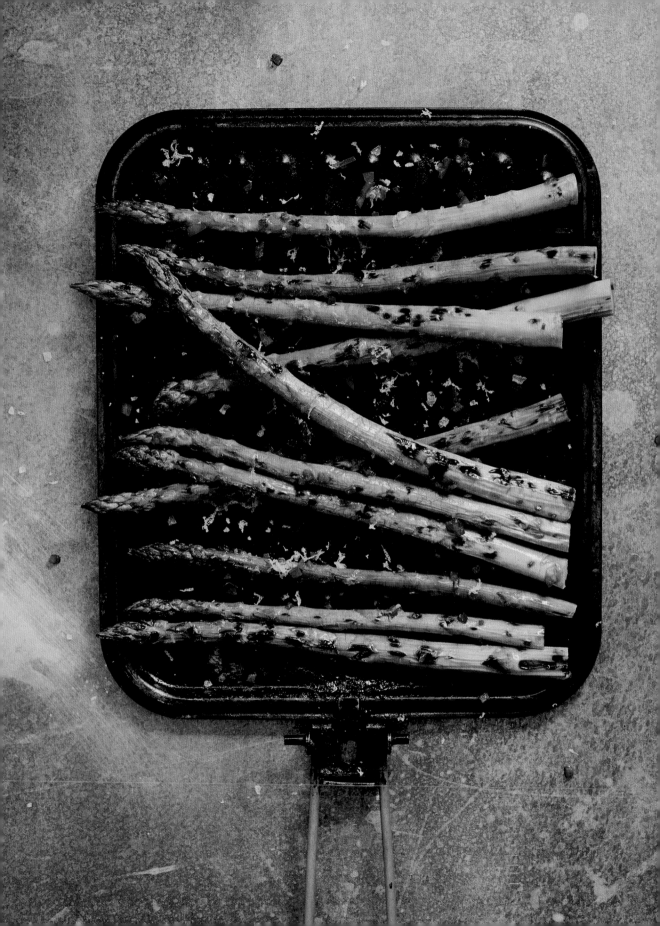

LEMON & CHILI GRIDDLED GREENS

This artfully simple side goes with anything. The keys are not to add any oil until the asparagus are cooked and to get really black char lines for depth of flavor, so try not to move the veggies around in the pan. This is a fast and easy side that makes the asparagus wonderfully tasty.

SERVES 2–3

7 oz asparagus
1 fresh red chili
2 tbsp olive oil
½ lemon
salt

Dry grill pan over highest heat

Bend the asparagus spears until they snap and throw the woody ends away | Lay them in the hot pan, perpendicular to the grill ridges | Leave for about 2–3 minutes for thin spears or up to 5 minutes for thick spears | Don't move them until they have developed deep black grill marks, then flip them over and repeat on the other side

Meanwhile, rip the stem from the chili, cut it in half lengthwise, and remove the seeds, if you prefer a milder flavor, and finely chop | Once the asparagus spears are charred on both sides, drizzle with the oil and scatter on the chopped chili | Squeeze the lemon over the veggies, catching the seeds in your other hand | Sprinkle with a pinch of salt, stir, and cook for another 60–90 seconds | Take off the heat and serve immediately

ULTIMATE BBQ COLESLAW

This is an awesome coleslaw. It feels fresh and healthy, but is also drenched in naughty BBQ sauce, which makes it incredibly indulgent. Serve inside the Big BOSH! Burger (see page 119) or as a side at a BBQ.

SERVES 6–8

1 large red cabbage (about 2 lb)
olive oil
⅔ cup BBQ sauce
1 onion
2 carrots
salt and black pepper

FOR THE DRESSING
3 limes, plus a little extra
scant 1 cup vegan mayonnaise
1 tsp English mustard, prepared
½ tsp hot sauce, optional
2 tsp salt
1 tsp black pepper
good pinch of cayenne pepper

Preheat oven to 350°F | Roasting pan | Pastry brush

Cut the cabbage in half, cut out and discard the core, then chop into about 8 pieces. Tip into a roasting pan | Brush the cabbage all over with oil and cover with the BBQ sauce | Season with salt and pepper | Put the roasting pan in the hot oven and cook for about 45 minutes, removing when the cabbage is nice and blackened, but not burned | Let it cool down for 10 minutes

Halve the limes for the dressing and squeeze the juice into a bowl, catching any seeds in your other hand | Add the rest of the dressing ingredients and stir to a smooth, well mixed consistency

Peel and finely slice the onion | Peel the carrots and slice them thinly using a vegetable peeler or sharp knife | When the cabbage is cool enough to handle, slice the pieces finely

Put all the veg in a serving bowl and pour the dressing over | Stir well, taste, and add more salt, pepper, or lime juice as desired

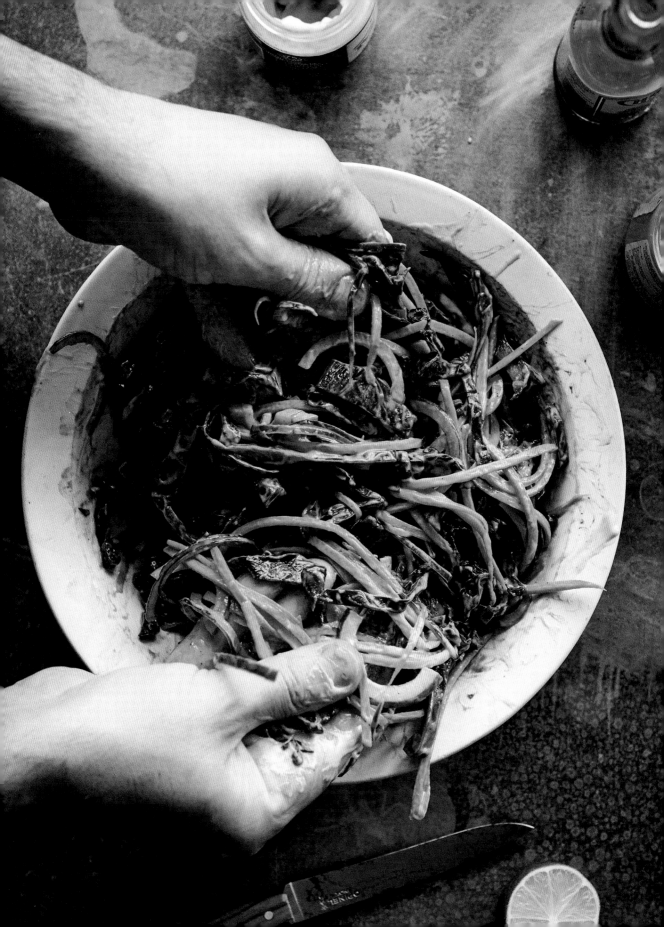

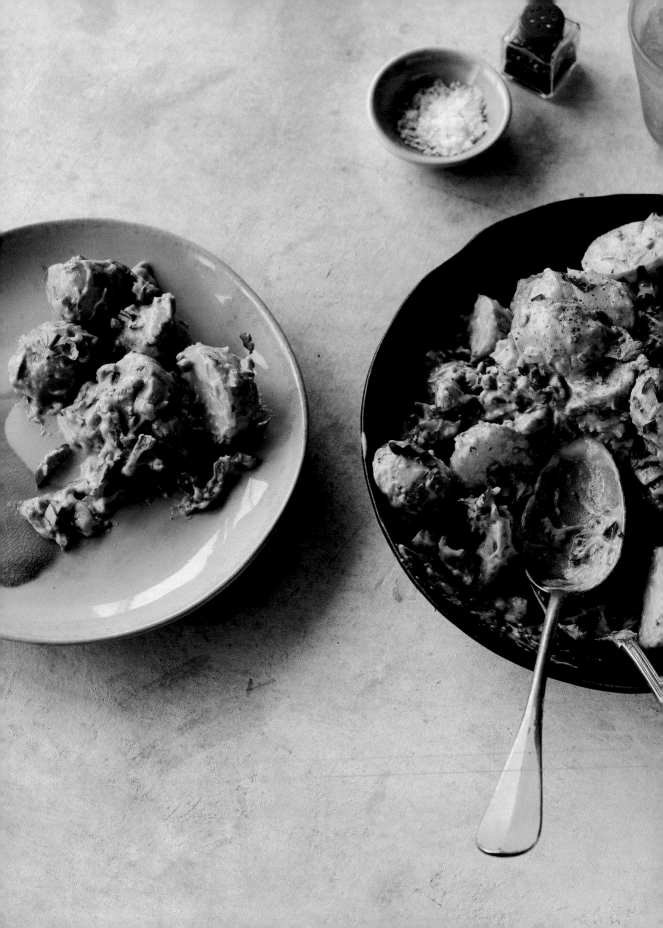

GUACAMOLE POTATO SALAD

This is a winning creation—it's creamy, rich, and luscious with a lime twist. This is the perfect side for a BBQ and brings back memories of childhood potato salads, but with a remixed, delicious Mexican flavor. This is a go-to dish of ours and we promise it will not disappoint.

SERVES 4–6

2¼ lb new potatoes
2 tbsp dairy-free butter or spread
1 lime
3 avocados
2 tbsp olive oil
¼ cup unsweetened plant-based milk
2 tbsp vegan mayonnaise
2 tsp garlic powder
2 tsp salt, plus a little extra
1 tsp black pepper
9 oz cherry tomatoes
1 large fresh red chili
½ red onion
1½ oz fresh cilantro

Large saucepan with a lid | Blender

Cut the potatoes into quarters (or halves if they're small) and put them in the saucepan | Fill the pan with cold water and add a large pinch of salt | Turn the heat to high and bring to a boil, then reduce the heat to low and simmer for 8–10 minutes, until the potatoes are cooked through | Drain and tip back into the pan | Add the dairy-free butter and stir so the potatoes are well covered, then set aside

Halve the lime and squeeze the juice into the blender | Halve and carefully pit the avocados by tapping the pit firmly with the heel of a knife so that it lodges in the pits, then twist and remove the pits | Scoop the avocado flesh into the blender | Add the olive oil, plant-based milk, vegan mayonnaise, garlic powder, salt, and pepper and whizz to a thick cream, adding a splash more plant-based milk if needed

Dice the cherry tomatoes | Rip the stem from the chili, cut it in half lengthwise, and remove the seeds, if you prefer a milder flavor, then finely chop | Peel and finely chop the onion | Put the chopped vegetables into a large serving bowl and add the dressing and potatoes | Chop the cilantro leaves and finely slice the stems and sprinkle into the bowl | Stir everything together so that it's well mixed, then enjoy!

FALAFEL BOSH! BOWL

This zingy, zesty salad with contrasting earthy falafel flavors
is the perfect reward for a gym visit or as an accompaniment
to a BBQ. You can make it ahead and, since it's so healthy, you
can really fill yourself up and still feel great. Feel free to sub
out the falafel if you just want a quick and easy Greek salad.

SERVES 4–6

3½ oz leafy salad leaves
1 lemon
small handful fresh cilantro leaves
handful fresh mint, optional

FOR THE HUMMUS
½ lemon
1 can (15 oz) chickpeas
3 tbsp aquafaba (water from
    chickpea can)
1½ tbsp tahini
1½ tbsp olive oil
1 garlic clove
1 tsp salt

FOR THE FALAFEL
2 cans (15 oz each) chickpeas
2 small red onions
3 garlic cloves
1 cup fresh cilantro leaves
1 cup fresh flat-leaf parsley leaves
generous ¾ cup chickpea flour
1½ tbsp harissa paste
2 tsp salt
1 tsp ground cumin
½ tsp black pepper
½ lemon
olive oil, for frying

FOR THE GREEK SALAD
½ cucumber
1¾ lb mixed tomatoes
½ small red onion
2½ oz pine nuts (or any nuts)
5 oz pitted black Kalamata olives
    (but any olives will do)
3 tbsp red wine vinegar
3 tbsp olive oil
1 tsp dried oregano
salt and black pepper

Food processor | Large frying pan | Small frying pan

First make the hummus | Cut the lemon in half and squeeze the juice
into the food processor, catching the seeds in your other hand | Add all
the rest of the ingredients and blend to a smooth paste | Scrape into a
bowl and set aside (there's no need to rinse the processor bowl)

Now make the falafel | Drain the chickpeas | Peel and finely chop the red
onions and garlic | Finely chop the cilantro and parsley | Put all the falafel
ingredients except for the oil and lemon in the food processor | Squeeze
the lemon juice into the processor, catching any seeds in your other
hand | Whizz to a thick paste

Using wet hands to stop the batter sticking, pick out small pieces of
falafel batter between your finger and thumb and create little balls
¾–1 inch in width (about the size of a large marble) until you've used
up all the batter

Put the large frying pan over high heat and add the olive oil | Add the balls
to the pan and cook for 2–3 minutes until golden all over, using a spatula
to flip them halfway through (you may need to do this in batches)

To make the salad, trim and slice the cucumber, cut the tomatoes into
wedges, and peel and thinly slice the onion | Set the small frying pan
over medium heat and put the pine nuts into the dry pan to toast for a
few minutes | Tip the chopped vegetables into a large bowl with the
toasted pine nuts and olives | Pour in the red wine vinegar and olive oil,
sprinkle with the oregano, and season with salt and pepper | Mix it all
together

Get out four to six big bowls and lay a few salad leaves into each one
| Fill each bowl with big helpings of Greek salad, hummus, and falafel
| Cut the lemon in half and squeeze over some juice, catching any seeds
in your other hand before serving with a sprinkling of fresh cilantro and
mint, if using

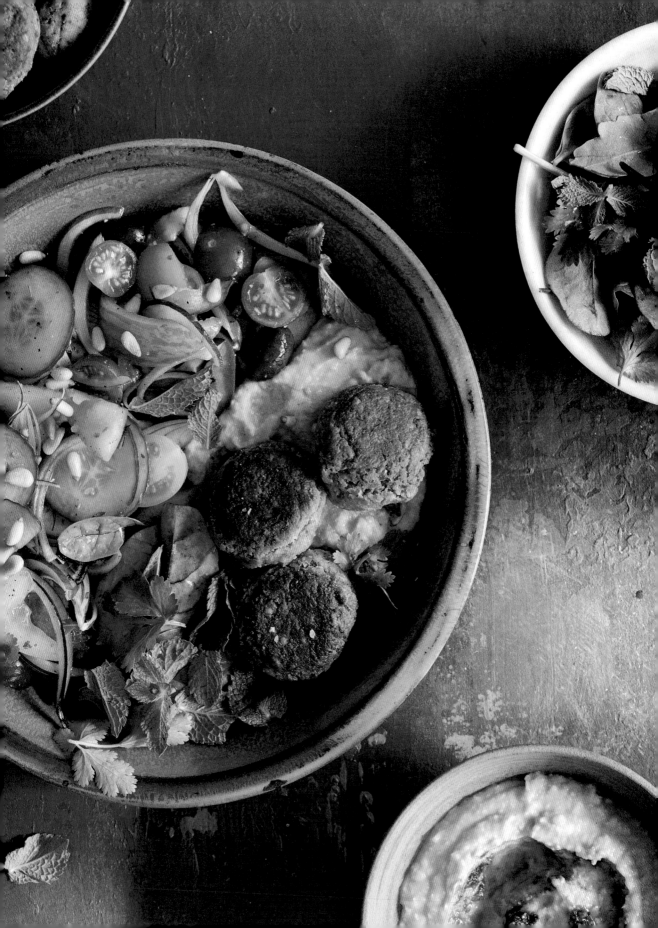

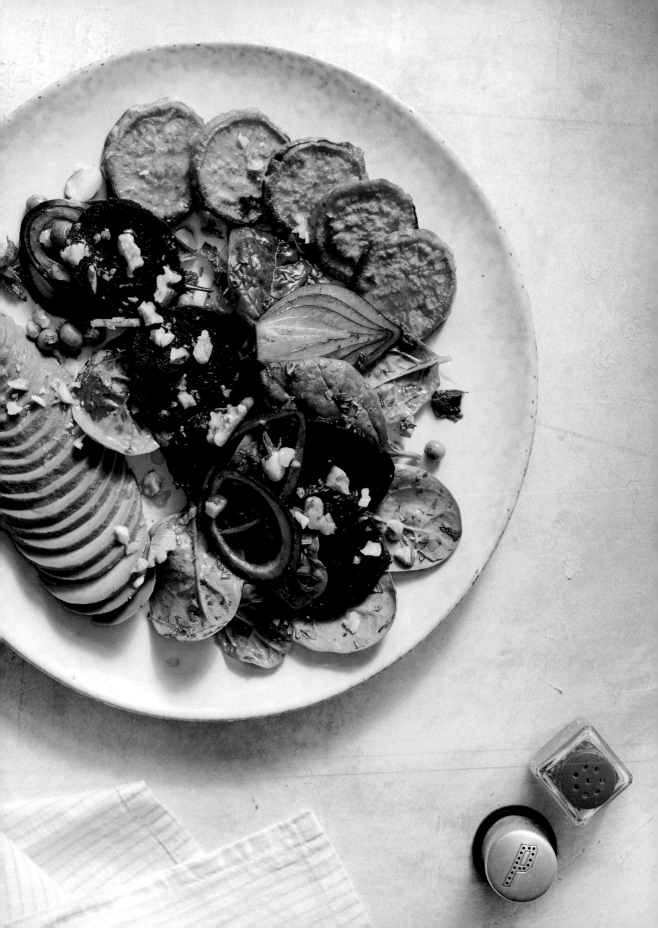

BEET, ONION & SWEET POTATO SALAD

We wanted a salad with Beet, Onion, Sweet potato, and Herbs (B.O.S.H., get it?). We love beets and were keen to base a salad around them. This is incredibly tasty and can be made even more filling by using two sweet potatoes or sprinkling some more nuts on top for a protein boost.

SERVES 4

1 sweet potato (2 if you're hungry)
4 garlic cloves
¼ cup + 2 tbsp olive oil
10 oz cooked beet
1 small red onion
3 tbsp white wine vinegar
2 tsp hot sauce
5 oz fresh or frozen peas
3½ oz baby spinach
large handful fresh cilantro leaves
large handful fresh mint leaves
2 medium avocados
handful mixed nuts
salt and black pepper

Preheat oven to 390°F | Baking sheet

Peel the sweet potato and cut it into ⅓-inch rounds | Lay them on the baking sheet along with 3 unpeeled garlic cloves | Pour on the 2 tablespoons of oil and sprinkle with salt and pepper | Put into the hot oven for 20 minutes until soft and charring slightly at the edges | Remove and set aside

Meanwhile, finely slice the beets and place them in a bowl | Peel and mince the onion | Peel the remaining garlic clove and finely slice half (use the other half for something else) | Add both to the beets | Pour on the white wine vinegar, the ¼ cup of oil, and the hot sauce | Mix well and leave to infuse while the sweet potato bakes

Put the peas into a small microwave-safe bowl, cover with a splash of water, and cook on full power for 4 minutes | Quickly drain and run under cold water to cool, then add to the large bowl | Add the spinach | Finely chop the cilantro and mint leaves and add to the bowl | Gently toss everything together

Just before you're ready to eat, halve and carefully pit the avocados by tapping the pits firmly with the heel of a knife so that it lodges in the pits. Twist and remove the pits | Run a spoon around the inside of the skin to scoop out the avocado halves, then slice finely, trying to keep the shape of the avocado halves

Divide the salad among serving plates | Put a neat line of sweet potato slices on each plate and add a small pile of avocado | Spoon the beets over the plate | Roughly chop the nuts and scatter them over and enjoy this delicious, healthy meal!

SATAY SWEET POTATO BOSH! BOWL

This powerful salad combines some of our favorite ingredients: satay sauce, hummus, and sweet potato. It's gluten-free, healthy, and delicious! Peanuts feature heavily in this staple and incredibly moreish satay sauce of ours. Filled with protein and healthy goodness, this dish will leave you satisfied for ages!

SERVES 2

1 large sweet potato (about 10 oz)
½ red onion
olive oil
1–2 tsp chili flakes
2 garlic cloves
generous 1 cup cooked quinoa
    (homemade or store-bought)
5 oz broccoli (about ½ medium head)
1 avocado
handful crushed nuts
⅔ cup hummus (store-bought
    or see page 199)
2 tbsp mixed seeds, to serve
salt and black pepper

FOR THE DRESSING

2 limes
¾-inch piece fresh ginger
1 garlic clove
1 fresh red chili
10 sprigs fresh cilantro
3 heaping tbsp good-quality
    crunchy peanut butter
1 tbsp soy sauce

Preheat oven to 350°F | Blender | Roasting pan

Cut the sweet potato into 1-inch chunks, keeping the skin | Cut the red onion half into quarters and place in the roasting pan with the sweet potato | Drizzle with some olive oil, sprinkle with the chili flakes, and season with a little salt and pepper | Crush the unpeeled garlic cloves by pressing down on them with the back of a knife and add to the roasting pan | Put the pan in the oven for 15 minutes

Heat the cooked quinoa in the microwave | Break the broccoli into bite-sized florets | Take the pan out of the oven and add the broccoli, mixing everything around with a wooden spoon | Put the roasting pan back in the oven and bake for 15 minutes longer, until the potatoes and broccoli are softened | Remove from the oven

Meanwhile, make the dressing | Zest the limes, cut them in half, and squeeze the juice into the blender, catching any seeds in your other hand | Peel the ginger by scraping off the skin with a spoon and roughly chop | Peel the garlic | Rip the stem from the chili, cut it in half lengthwise, and remove the seeds, if you prefer a milder dressing | Roughly chop the cilantro | Add all the ingredients for the dressing to the blender and whizz it all up | Test for consistency, adding spoonfuls of water until it's runny enough to pour over the salad

Halve and carefully pit the avocado by tapping the pit firmly with the heel of a knife so that it lodges in the pit, then twist and remove the pit | Run a spoon around the inside of the skin to scoop out the avocado halves, then slice

Divide the quinoa between two serving bowls | Arrange the roasted vegetables and nuts on the top | Add a large dollop of hummus and the avocado slices to the bowls | Drizzle a little dressing over the top of each and serve the rest on the side before sprinkling with seeds to serve

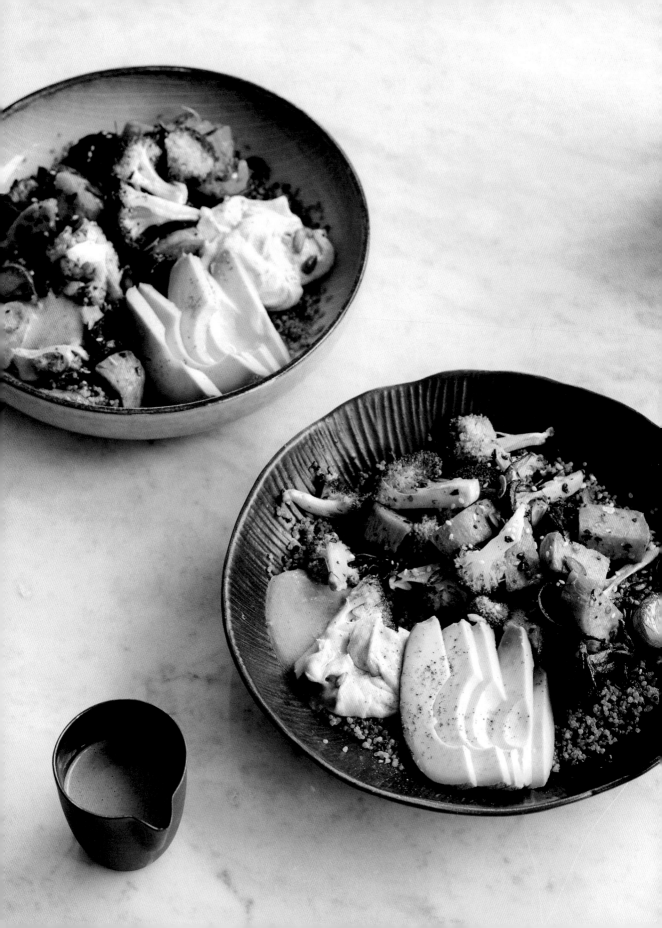

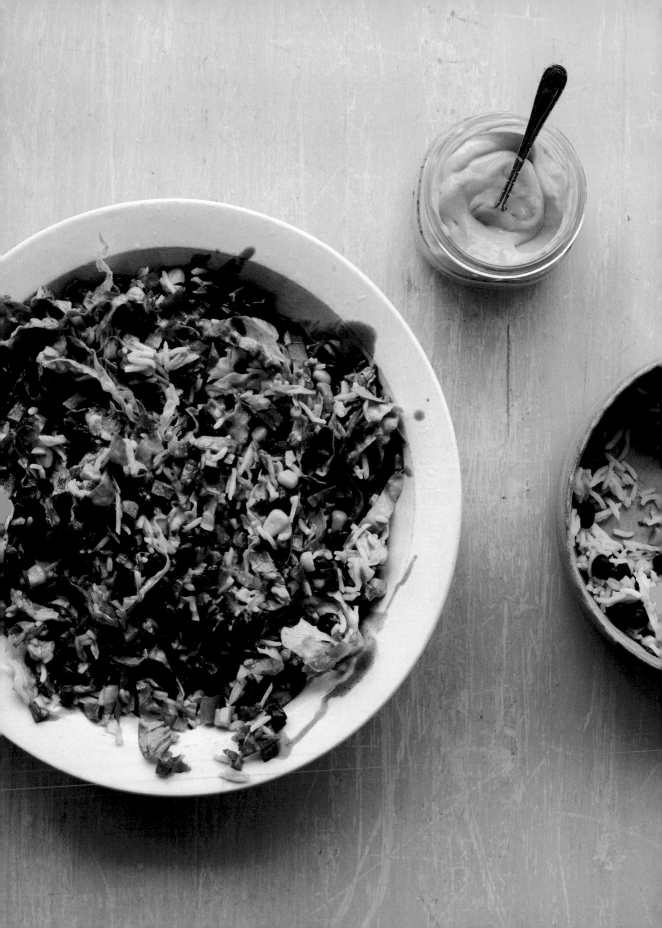

SOUTHWEST BOSH! BOWL

This was inspired by our desire to create the deliciousness of a burrito without the tortilla. It's a great source of protein and contains all your essential amino acids, making it a perfect post-workout meal for spring or summer. Fiery, citrusy, sweet, and fresh, it's an orchestra of healthy goodness. Plus, avocados—need we say more?

SERVES 2–4

1 cup cooked basmati rice (store-bought or Perfectly Boiled Rice, see page 207)
1 can (15 oz) black beans
1 can (7 oz) corn
2 large tomatoes
½ red bell pepper
½ small red onion
2 small avocados
1 lime
½ fresh green chili
1 tbsp olive oil
⅔ cup unsweetened plant-based milk
1 tsp maple syrup
½ tsp garlic powder
1 little gem lettuce
1¾ oz fresh cilantro
hot sauce, to serve
salt and black pepper

Medium saucepan | Blender

Tip the cooked rice into a mixing bowl, fluff it with a fork and transfer to a serving bowl

Drain the black beans and corn and add them to the rice

Halve the tomatoes, cut out the seeds, and finely dice | Trim any stem and seeds from the bell pepper and finely dice | Peel and finely dice the onion | Add the diced vegetables to the rice and fold together

Halve and carefully pit the avocados by tapping the pits firmly with the heel of a knife so that it lodges in the pits, then twist and remove the pits | Scoop the flesh into the blender | Cut the lime in half and squeeze in most of the juice, catching any seeds in your other hand | Rip the stem from the chili, cut it in half lengthwise, and remove the seeds, if you prefer a milder flavor | Add the chili, olive oil, plant-based milk, maple syrup, and garlic powder to the blender and whizz to a creamy sauce with a thick drizzling consistency, adding a splash more plant-based milk if necessary | Taste and adjust the seasoning as needed

Finely slice the lettuce | Chop the cilantro leaves and finely chop the stems | Add the lettuce and cilantro to the rice | Pour on the avocado dressing and stir everything together | Check the seasoning and add salt, pepper, or remaining lime juice to taste

Spoon into bowls to serve, drizzled with a little hot sauce

THE BEST-DRESSED BOSH! BOWL

The combination of balsamic, fennel, and garlic here lends a unique flavor to the roasted veggies—it's one of the most delicious ways to eat loads of goodness in one go. The dressing would suit any vegetables; just keep timing in mind to ensure they're properly cooked. Great as a light lunch, starter, or BBQ side.

SERVES 3–6

1 onion
4 garlic cloves
1 fresh red chili
1 tbsp fennel seeds
¼ cup olive oil, plus extra for drizzling
¼ cup balsamic vinegar,
    plus extra for drizzling
1 tbsp maple syrup
3 tbsp tomato paste
1¼ cups cooked puy lentils
12 oz butternut squash
1 fennel bulb
7 oz cherry tomatoes
1 yellow bell pepper
1 red bell pepper
1 zucchini
1 avocado
3½ oz baby spinach or kale
scant cup fresh flat-leaf parsley leaves
salt and black pepper

Preheat oven to 350°F | Medium saucepan over medium heat | Roasting pan

Peel the onion | Peel the garlic | Rip the stem from the chili, then cut it in half lengthwise and remove the seeds if you prefer a milder flavor | Finely chop the onion, garlic, chili, and fennel seeds | Spoon into the saucepan and add the ¼ cup of olive oil, balsamic vinegar, maple syrup, and tomato paste | Stir for 5 minutes, then add the cooked lentils | Stir to combine, remove from the heat, and set aside

Peel the squash, cut it in half, and remove the seeds, then cut into ¾-inch chunks | Tip into a roasting pan, drizzle with a little olive oil, season, and put the pan in the hot oven for 15 minutes, then remove

Meanwhile, trim the fennel bulb, remove the core, and cut into ⅓-inch wedges | Halve the tomatoes | Cut the bell peppers in half, cut out the stems and seeds | Trim the ends of the zucchini | Cut the pepper and zucchini into ⅓-inch pieces | Add the fennel, zucchini, peppers, and tomatoes to the roasting pan with the squash and drizzle over a little more oil | Return to the oven to cook for 15 minutes, until tender

While the vegetables are roasting, halve and carefully pit the avocado by tapping the pit firmly with the heel of a knife so that it lodges in the pit, then twist and remove the pit | Run a spoon around the inside of the skin to scoop out the avocado halves and cut into chunks | Wash and lightly chop the spinach or kale and roughly chop the parsley leaves

Remove the roasted veggies from the oven and tip into a serving bowl with the avocado, spinach or kale, parsley, and lentils | Stir and serve

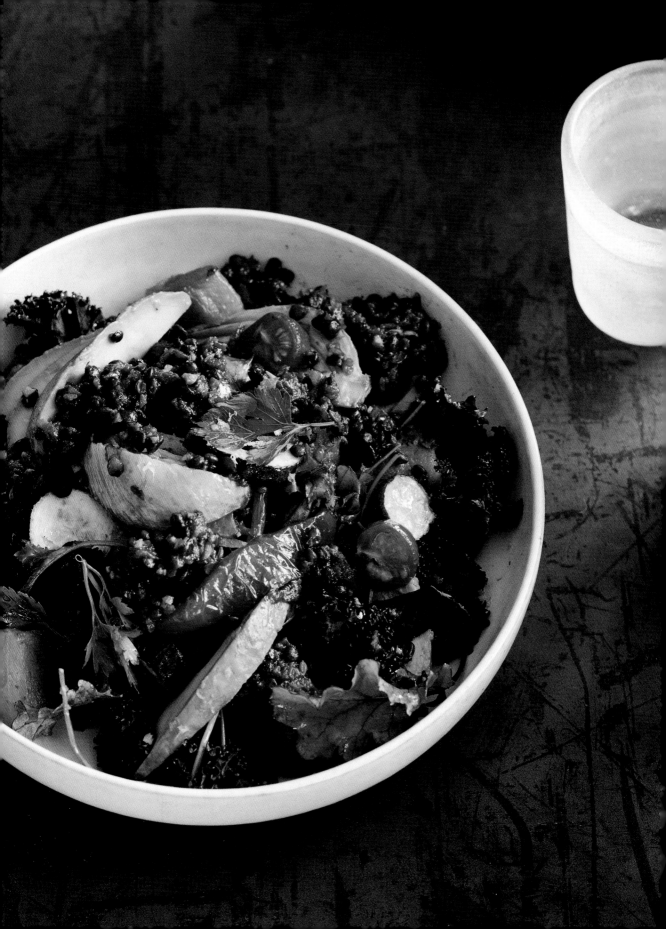

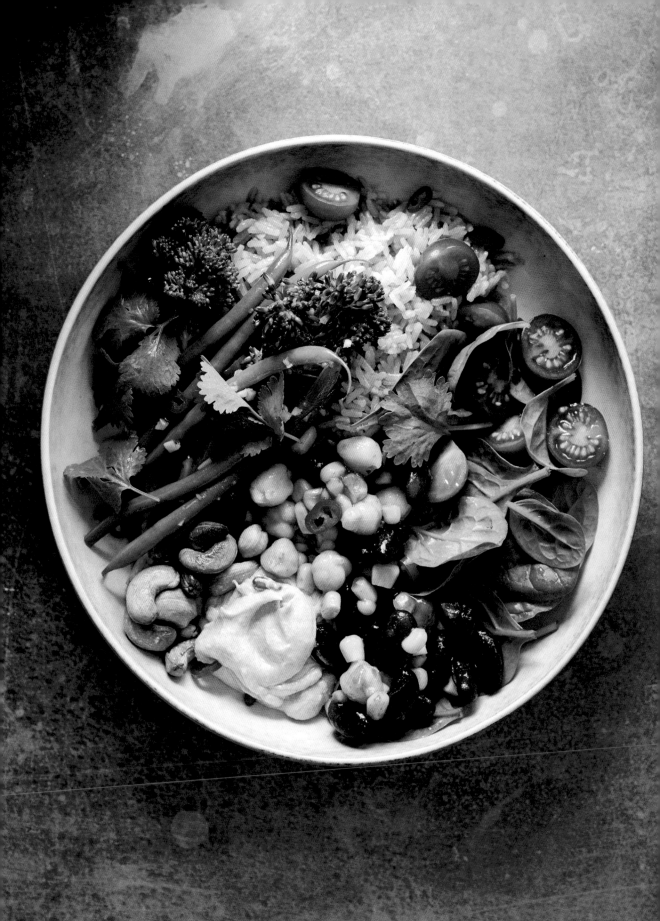

THE BIG GREEN BOSH! BOWL

This delicious dish is perfect post-gym fuel. It looks like a lot of food, but you'll wolf down the healthy greens and delicious dressing. Double up the recipe for a week's worth of turbo-sized lunches. This clever recipe uses the rice water to steam the veggies, so it's easy to cook and there's less cleanup.

SERVES 2

1 mug brown rice (about 1 cup)
2 mugs water (about 2 cups)
4 oz broccolini
2 oz green beans
1¼ cups canned mixed beans
    (or any bean, such as kidney beans)
1 fresh red chili
1 lemon
2 oz baby spinach
12 cherry tomatoes
2½ oz cashews
⅓ cup hummus (store-bought
    or see page 199)
handful fresh cilantro leaves
sriracha or other hot sauce, to serve
salt

FOR THE DRESSING
1 garlic clove
¾-inch piece fresh ginger
1 tbsp olive oil
1 tsp toasted sesame oil
1 tbsp soy sauce

Medium saucepan with a lid over medium-high heat | Boiling water | Steamer insert or metal colander

Fill a mug with brown rice, pour it into a sieve, and rinse with cold water for 30 seconds | Use the same mug to measure twice as much boiling water into the hot pan | Add a little salt | When the water returns to a boil, add the rice, put the lid on, stir, and cook for 20 minutes

Meanwhile, trim the bottoms from the broccolini | Top and tail the green beans

Next, make the dressing | Peel and finely chop the garlic | Peel the ginger by scraping off the skin with a spoon, chop, and put in a mug with the garlic | Pour in the olive oil, sesame oil, and soy sauce and stir

After 20 minutes, take the lid off the rice and put a steamer insert or heatproof colander on top of the pan | Add the green beans and broccoli and pour over half the dressing | Put a big lid on top of the insert or colander and set the timer for 5 minutes, then check the veg and rice are done; if not, cook for a little longer | Once everything is cooked, turn off the heat and leave the lid off the pan

Drain half the can of mixed beans (use the other half another time) | Rip the stem from the chili, cut it in half lengthwise, and remove the seeds if you prefer a milder flavor, then finely slice | Drain the rice if necessary | Cut the lemon in half

To assemble, divide the spinach between the bowls, followed by the mixed beans, steamed veggies, rice, and cherry tomatoes | Pile the cashews on top of the salad and spoon on a large dollop of hummus | Squeeze on the juice of the lemon, catching any seeds in your other hand

Drizzle the rest of the dressing over the top and sprinkle with the cilantro leaves and chili | Finish by squeezing a tablespoon of sriracha or hot sauce over everything

MAKE YOUR OWN BOSH! BOWLS

BOSH! bowls are protein-filled bowls of deliciousness. They are typically filled with plant-based proteins, green veg, and a grain of some kind. They're perfect for after the gym, or just for feeding your hungry belly during a busy day. You can quickly knock them together with whatever you have in the fridge, just cover each of these bases to ensure tastiness and healthiness!

1. **Choose your grain**
   Brown or white rice
   Couscous
   Quinoa
   Rice noodles
   Soba noodles
   Whole wheat noodles

2. **Add your protein:**
   Black beans
   Butter beans or lima beans
   Kidney beans
   Lentils
   Pinto beans
   Seitan
   Tempeh
   Tofu

3. **Trim and finely slice the vegetables, then roast or steam them and add to the bowl**
   Asparagus
   Beets
   Broccoli
   Carrots
   Green beans
   Mushrooms
   Onions
   Peppers
   Sweet potatoes
   Zucchini

4. **Finely slice some raw veg and add straight to the bowl and stir everything together**
   Avocado
   Chili peppers
   Corn
   Cucumber
   Greens
   Kale
   Lettuce
   Peppers
   Scallions
   Spinach

5. **Chop the herbs, chuck into the bowl, and mix through**
   Basil
   Chives
   Cilantro
   Dill
   Mint
   Parsley
   Tarragon

6. **Roughly chop some nuts or seeds, or leave whole and add raw or toasted and scatter over the top**
   Blanched almonds
   Cashews
   Chia seeds
   Flaxseeds
   Hazelnuts
   Macadamia nuts
   Mixed nuts
   Peanuts
   Pecans
   Pine nuts
   Pumpkin seeds
   Sesame seeds
   Walnuts

7. **Choose your dressing and drizzle it over**
   Baba Ganoush (see page 193)
   Balsamic vinegar
   Hummus (see page 199)
   Lemon juice
   Mango chutney
   Mustard
   Olive oil
   Olive Tapenade (see page 192)
   Proper Spanish Aioli (see page 192)
   Rich Satay Sauce (see page 193)
   Soy or coconut yogurt-based dressing
   Soy sauce

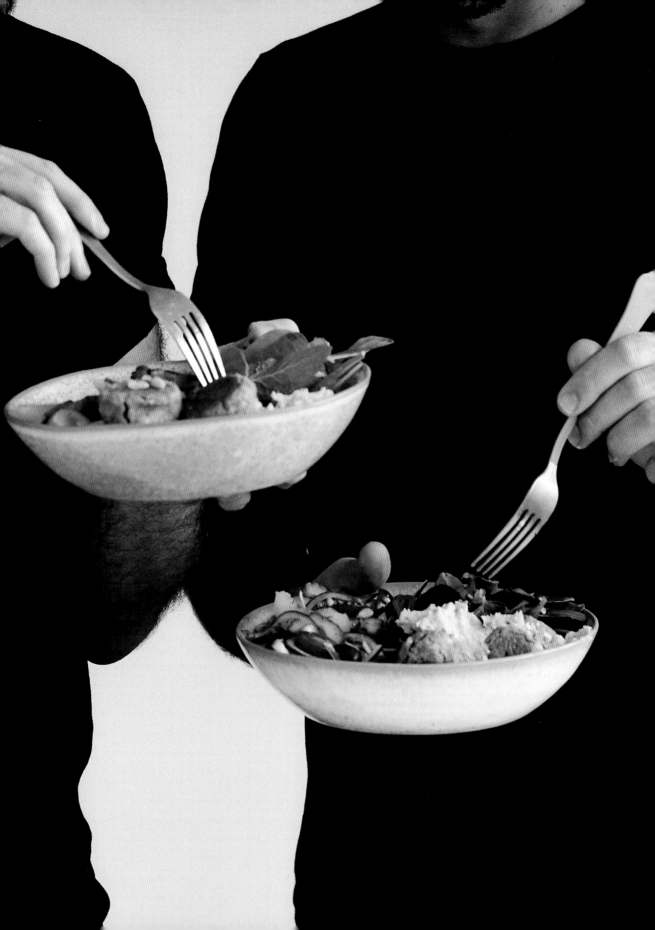

05

SMALL PLATES & SHARERS

Pimp out your mini-bites
With delicious sharing plates
For sides or tapas

CAULIFLOWER BUFFALO WINGS

These delicious wings taste naughty but are actually healthy, since they're baked. The spices are gorgeously deep and the panko breadcrumbs give a crunchy coating that contrasts nicely with the smooth cauliflower. It's the perfect starter or dish to share with friends. We promise, you'll love it.

SERVES 2–4

1 large head of cauliflower
1 cup + 2 tbsp all-purpose flour
1¼ cups unsweetened plant-based milk
2 tsp garlic powder
1 tsp onion powder
1 tsp ground cumin
1 tsp paprika
½ tsp salt
¼ tsp black pepper
1 cup panko breadcrumbs
8 tbsp dairy-free butter or spread
¾ cup Buffalo hot sauce

FOR THE RANCH SAUCE

5 oz cashews
⅔ cup unsweetened plant-based milk
1 tbsp lemon juice
2 tsp garlic powder
¾ tsp salt
¼ tsp black pepper
handful fresh parsley
4 chives

Preheat oven to 350°F | Line 2 baking sheets | Small saucepan of boiling water over high heat | Food processor or blender

Add the cashews to the pan of boiling water and boil for 15 minutes, then drain and run under cold water to cool slightly

Meanwhile, break the cauliflower into florets and cut the stem into bite-sized pieces

Put the flour, plant-based milk, garlic powder, onion powder, cumin, paprika, salt, and pepper into a bowl and whisk to a batter | Pour the panko breadcrumbs into another bowl and rub them between your thumb and fingers to break into slightly smaller breadcrumbs

Tip the cauliflower into the batter and toss to coat | Transfer to the bowl of breadcrumbs, a few pieces at a time, and toss gently until well coated | Spread the cauliflower pieces over the lined baking sheets and bake for 20 minutes

Meanwhile, melt the dairy-free butter in the microwave and stir in the hot sauce

After 20 minutes, remove the pans from the oven, drizzle with the butter/hot sauce, and carefully roll the cauliflower around until the pieces are fully coated | Put the pans back in the oven for 20–25 minutes, until a sharp knife glides into the thickest parts of the cauliflower and the outsides are really golden brown and crispy | Remove from the oven

While the cauliflower is cooking, put all the ingredients for the ranch sauce except for the herbs into the food processor or blender and whizz for 1–2 minutes until smooth and creamy | Transfer to a serving bowl | Finely chop the parsley and chives and add most of them to the sauce, reserving a little for garnish

Serve the cauliflower wings while they're still hot on a serving plate, sprinkled with the remaining herbs and with the ranch sauce on the side

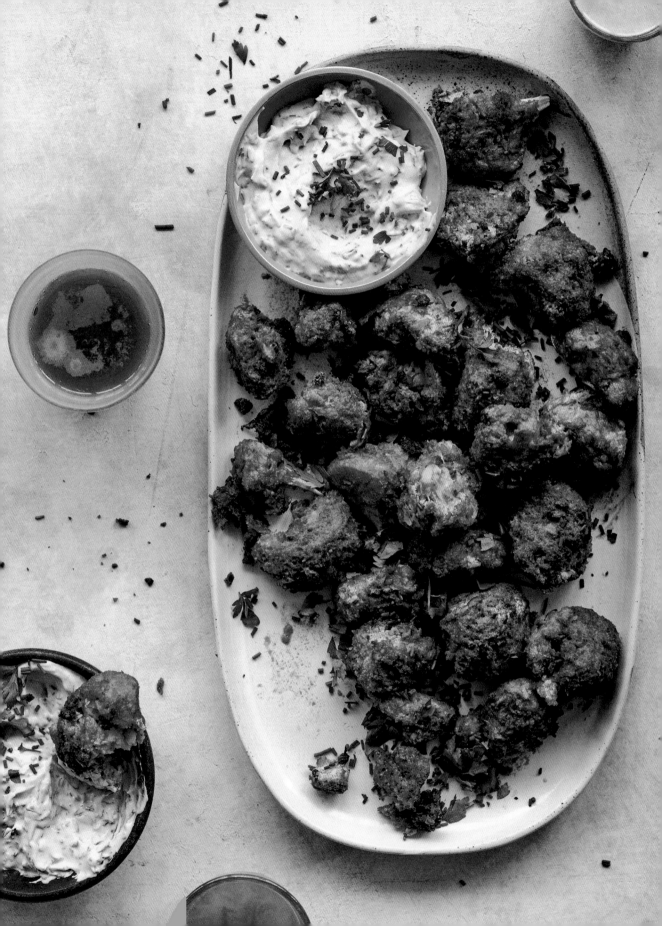

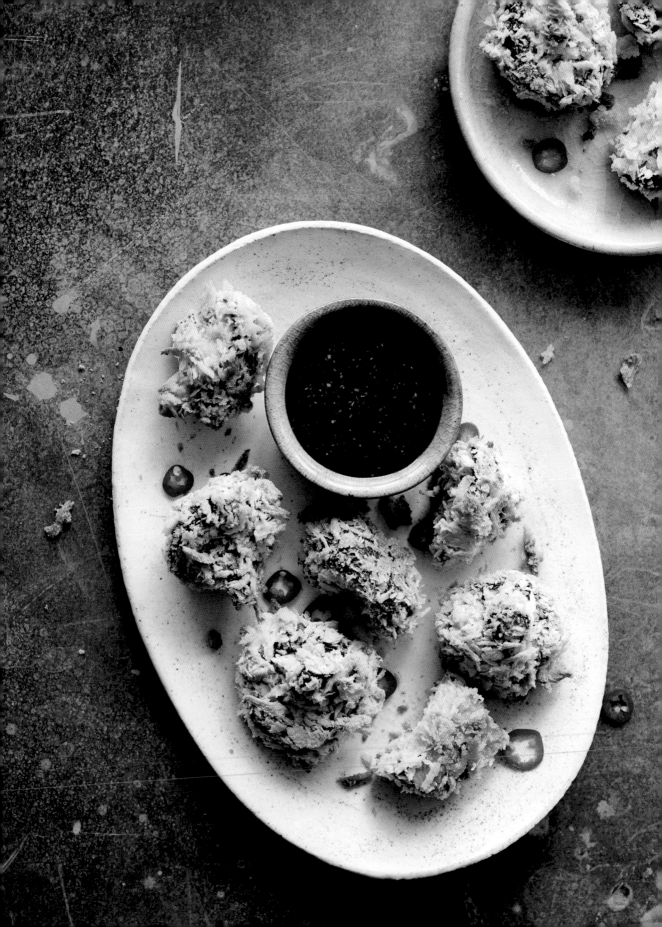

SHIITAKE TERIYAKI DIPPERS

Once you've had your fill of these dippers, there won't
be mush-room left in your belly for anything else (ahem)!
They are crunchy and crispy, sweet and sticky, deliciously
mushroomy inside and covered by a sumptuous sauce.
A healthy bake with the luxurious feeling of a deep-fry,
this is great nibble-fodder.

SERVES 2

5 tsp soy sauce
9 tbsp water
½ tsp ground ginger
½ tsp garlic powder
2½ tbsp brown sugar
1 tbsp cornstarch
9 oz shiitake or wild mushrooms
1¼ cups panko breadcrumbs

FOR THE BATTER
¾ cup + 2 tbsp unsweetened plant-
   based milk
¾ cup + 2 tbsp all-purpose flour
2 tsp garlic powder
2 tsp onion salt

**Preheat oven to 390°F | Line 2 baking sheets | Small saucepan over
medium heat**

Put the soy sauce, 7 tbsp of the water, the ground ginger, garlic powder,
and sugar into the hot pan and simmer gently until the sugar dissolves

Put the cornstarch and remaining 2 tbsp water into a glass and stir with a
fork until there are no lumps | Add to the pan, turn up the heat, and
bring to a boil, stirring as you go | Reduce the heat and simmer for
2–3 minutes, stirring frequently, until the sauce is syrupy and viscous |
Pour into a bowl and set aside

Put all the ingredients for the batter into a mixing bowl and stir to combine
| Cut any large mushrooms in half and add all the mushrooms to the
batter to coat thoroughly

Put the panko breadcrumbs into a large bowl

One by one, roll the battered mushrooms in the breadcrumbs and place
them on the lined baking sheets | Put the pans in the oven and bake for
18–20 minutes, until the mushrooms are golden brown and crispy
| Remove from the oven, put them in a serving bowl, and serve with the
teriyaki sauce

POPCORN FALAFEL

We call these "nom nom balls," and they are unacceptably good for a dippy dinner party. Crispy, crunchy, and moreish, you may need to make double helpings (served with hummus, obviously). They are the best dipping food we have ever tasted, good as a snack, great in pita, and an audacious way to enjoy a Middle Eastern staple!

SERVES 6–8

1 small red onion

3 garlic cloves

2 cans (15 oz each) chickpeas

1¾ cups all-purpose flour, plus a little extra

1 cup fresh cilantro leaves

1 cup fresh parsley

2 tsp harissa paste

1 tsp ground cumin

2 tsp salt

1 tsp pepper

1 lemon

1⅔ cups panko breadcrumbs

1 cup unsweetened plant-based milk

3 cups vegetable oil, for frying

Double batch of Classic Hummus (see page 199), to serve

Line a large bowl with a clean kitchen towel | Food processor | Large deep saucepan | Line a plate with paper towels

Peel the onion and the garlic | Drain and rinse the chickpeas and tip them into the bowl lined with a kitchen towel | Pat the chickpeas dry to remove as much moisture as possible

Put the onion, garlic, and chickpeas into the food processor | Add ¾ cup of the flour, the cilantro, parsley, harissa, cumin, 1 teaspoon of the salt, and ½ teaspoon of the pepper | Cut the lemon in half and squeeze in the juice, catching any seeds with your other hand | Whizz to a thick paste that's not too sticky (if it seems too wet, add another tablespoon or two of flour)

With lightly floured hands, take teaspoons of the mixture at a time and roll them into ¾-inch balls about the size of large marbles

Put the panko breadcrumbs into a bowl | Put the remaining 1 cup flour, the plant-based milk, and the remaining salt and pepper into a bowl and stir them together until you have a thick, creamy batter | Dip 2 or 3 balls at a time into the batter, shake off any excess, and transfer them to the bowl of breadcrumbs, rolling them around until they are completely coated | Repeat until all of the balls are coated

Pour the vegetable oil into the large deep saucepan so that it comes no more than two-thirds up the side of the pan | Place the pan over medium heat | When a small piece of bread dropped into the pan turns golden brown after 60 seconds, you are ready to go

Fry the falafels in batches of 10 for 3–4 minutes, then turn them over and fry for a further 3 minutes, until deep golden brown and crisp | Remove from the pan with a slotted spoon and drain on the paper towels to remove the excess oil | Serve with hummus

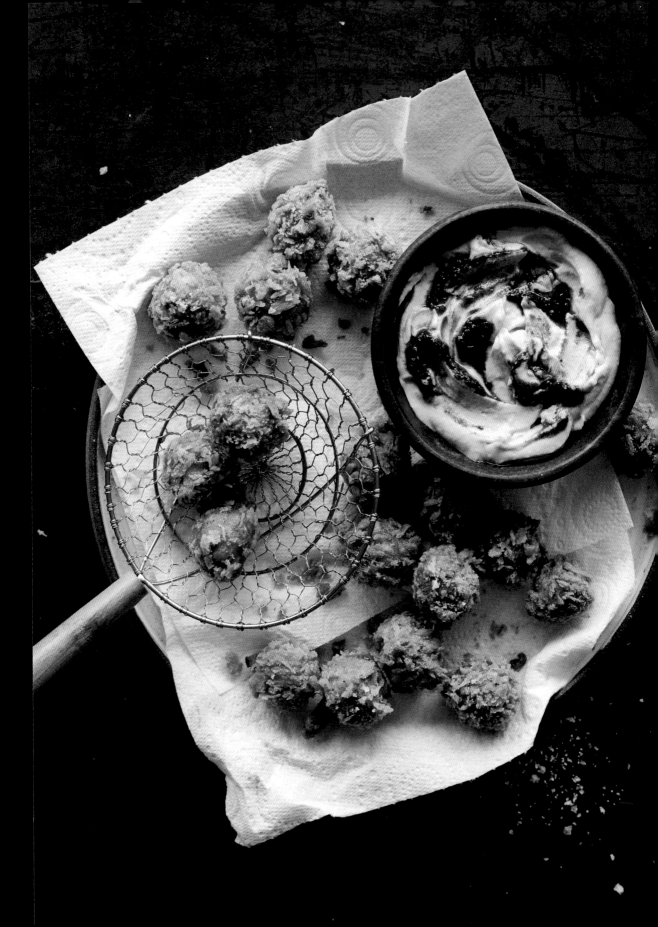

MAKI SUSHI ROLLS

These maki rolls are sushi with a BOSH! twist. Imagine the most delicious California rolls you can think of. The flavors really pop when these are combined with a bit of soy sauce, ginger, and wasabi. To make exotic DIY lunches, wrap them in foil and take them to work with you for the ultimate maki roll treat. Turn the page for inspiration.

GUACA MAKI ROLLS

SERVES 4

1½ cups sushi rice
¼ cup rice vinegar
2 tbsp superfine sugar
½ tsp salt
½ cucumber
1 carrot
2 scallions
1 avocado
4 sheets sushi nori
2 cups guacamole (store-bought or see page 194)
soy sauce, to serve
wasabi, to serve
pickled ginger, to serve, optional

Large saucepan | Small saucepan over medium-high heat | Large baking sheet | Sushi mat

Cook the sushi rice in the large saucepan, according to the package directions and ensuring that it is dry and sticky with no excess water once cooked

Pour the rice vinegar, sugar, and salt into the small saucepan and heat until the sugar has completely dissolved | Let the mixture cool to room temperature and then pour it over the cooked rice, gently stirring until all the liquid has been absorbed | Transfer the rice to a large baking sheet, spread it out to help it cool quicker, and leave it to cool to room temperature, by which point it should be dry but sticky

Cut the cucumber in half lengthwise and scoop out the watery seeds, then cut it into thin matchsticks roughly the same length as the width of a nori sheet | Trim the carrot and scallions and cut into matches the same size as the cucumber | Remove the avocado pit by tapping it firmly with the heel of a knife so that it lodges in the pit, then twist and remove the pit | Run a spoon around the inside of the skin to scoop out the avocado flesh, then slice into matchsticks

Take a nori sheet and lay it on the sushi mat, shiny side down | Spoon a quarter of the prepared rice onto the nori sheet, then dip the spoon in water and use it to spread out the rice to make a thin even layer, leaving a ⅓-inch gap at the farthest end of the nori sheet | Spread a very thin layer of guacamole on top of the rice | Lay a quarter of the avocado, scallion, carrot, and cucumber across the rice at the edge closest to you

Dip your finger in water and wet the exposed strip of nori | Use the bamboo mat to help you roll up the sushi from the end nearest you, compacting it as you go to ensure it is even and tightly wrapped | Repeat to make 4 sushi logs

To serve, use a very sharp wet knife to cut the rolls into bite-sized pieces, cleaning the knife with water after each cut (alternatively, leave them whole and eat as you would a wrap) | Serve with soy sauce, wasabi, and ginger, if using, on the side

SATAY MAKI ROLLS

SERVES 4

1½ cups sushi rice
¼ cup rice vinegar
2 tbsp superfine sugar
½ tsp salt
½ cucumber
1 carrot
2 scallions
1 avocado
Rich Satay Sauce (see page 193)
4 sheets sushi nori
soy sauce, to serve
wasabi, to serve
pickled ginger, to serve, optional

**Large saucepan | Small saucepan over medium-high heat
| Large baking sheet | Sushi mat**

Prepare the rice and vegetables as for Guaca Maki Rolls (see opposite)

Loosen the satay sauce by adding about 3–4 tablespoons water so that it's thick enough to hold its shape when rolled, but not too thick to spread

Take a nori sheet and lay it on the sushi mat, shiny side down | Spoon a quarter of the prepared rice onto the nori sheet, then dip the spoon in water and use it to spread out the rice to make a thin even layer, leaving a ⅓-inch gap at the farthest end of the nori sheet | Spread a very thin layer of satay sauce on top of the rice | Lay a quarter of the avocado, scallion, carrot, and cucumber across the rice at the edge closest to you

Dip your finger in water and wet the exposed strip of nori | Use the bamboo mat to help you roll up the sushi from the end nearest you, compacting it as you go to ensure it is even and tightly wrapped | Repeat to make 4 sushi logs

To serve, use a very sharp wet knife to cut the rolls into bite-sized pieces, cleaning the knife with water after each cut (alternatively, leave them whole and eat as you would a wrap) | Serve immediately with soy sauce, wasabi, and ginger, if using, on the side

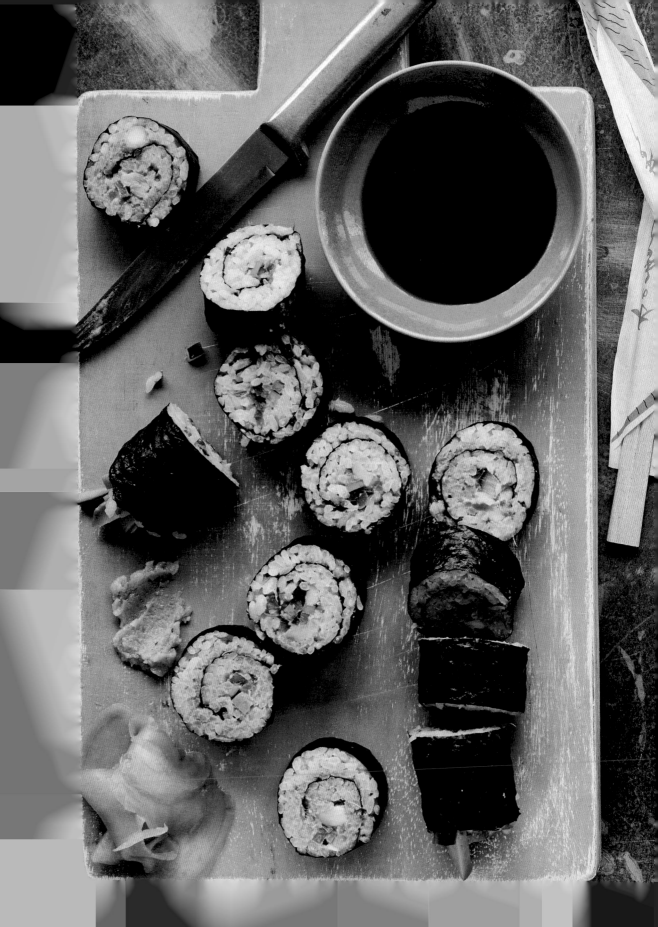

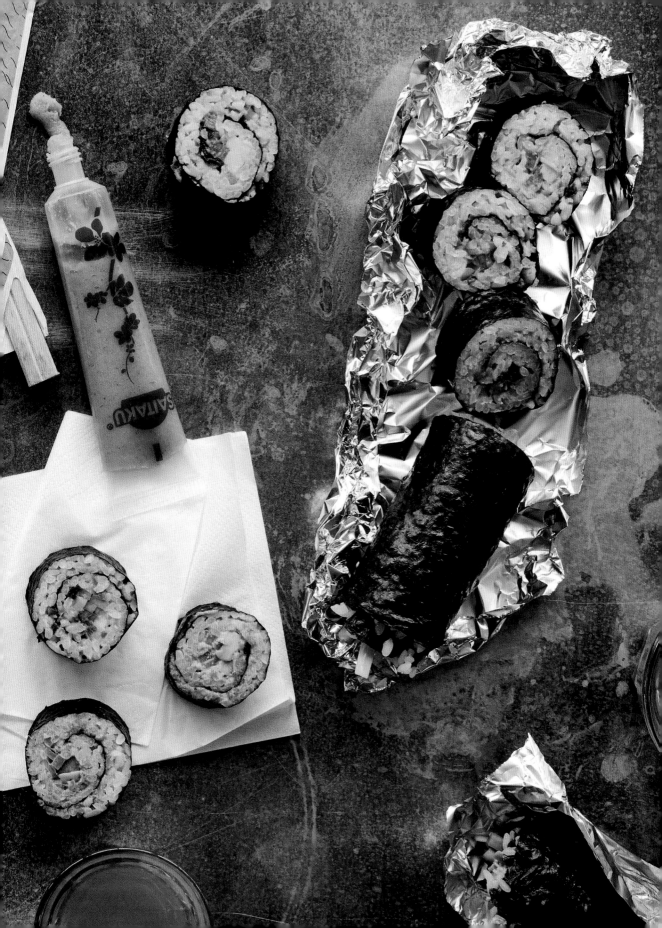

BANGIN' VEGGIE KEBABS

These are delicious and very good for you! The marinades are super quick to put together; if you don't have a blender, chop and mix in a big bowl until you get the right consistency. This is a great one for making in advance, since the marinades and veggies can be stored in the fridge. These go so well with a dipping sauce, and are perfect for a quick meal or BBQ. See them in their glory on page 180.

MAKES 8

2 red, orange, green, or yellow bell
   peppers
1 red onion
1 zucchini
1 eggplant
5 oz cherry tomatoes
9 oz mushrooms
Rich Satay, Spicy Shashlik, or Asian BBQ
   marinade (see opposite)

Preheat oven to 350°F | Blender | Small sheet pan | Wooden skewers, soaked

Cut the bell peppers in half and cut out the stem and seeds | Peel the onion | Trim the zucchini and eggplant | Cut all the vegetables into 1-inch chunks, put them in a big bowl, and cover them with your chosen marinade | Stir everything together until it's really well mixed

Thread the marinated vegetables onto the wooden skewers, leaving 1¼ inches free at either end | Lay the skewers across the sheet pan, resting each end on the edges so that the vegetables are suspended above the bottom (as if they're being spit-roasted)

Put the pan in the hot oven and roast for 20–25 minutes, until the vegetables are cooked through, deeply caramelized, and slightly crispy on the outside

MARINADES

Blender

Prepare your ingredients and then put them all into the blender | Whizz to a smooth paste

ASIAN BBQ

MAKES A GENEROUS ¾ CUP

2 fresh red chilies, stemmed
6 garlic cloves, peeled
1-inch piece fresh ginger, peeled
⅔ cup fresh cilantro leaves
½ tsp black pepper
¼ cup agave syrup
2 tbsp white wine vinegar
2 tbsp soy sauce

SPICY SHASHLIK

MAKES 1 CUP

2 large red chilies, stemmed
2 green bird's eye chilies, stemmed
6 garlic cloves, peeled
2-inch piece fresh ginger, peeled
2 tbsp sunflower oil
2 tsp ground cumin
1 tsp ground coriander
1 tsp garam masala
½ tsp ground turmeric
2 tsp smoked paprika
½ tsp chili powder
small handful fresh cilantro
2 tbsp tamarind paste
2 tbsp cornstarch
¼ cup white wine vinegar
¼ cup plain soy yogurt
1 tsp sea salt
¼ tsp black pepper

RICH SATAY

MAKES ¾ CUP

juice of 2 limes
1 fresh red chili, stemmed
1 garlic clove, peeled
¾-inch piece fresh ginger, peeled
⅔ cup fresh cilantro
generous ½ cup good-quality crunchy
    peanut butter
1 tbsp soy sauce
1–2 tbsp water, optional, to
    achieve runny consistency

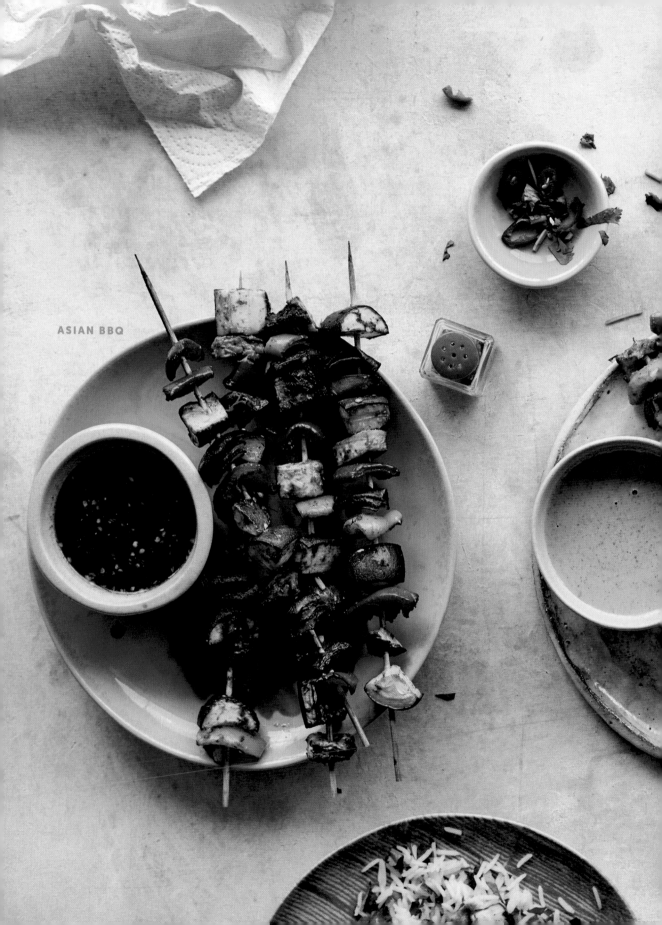

ASIAN BBQ

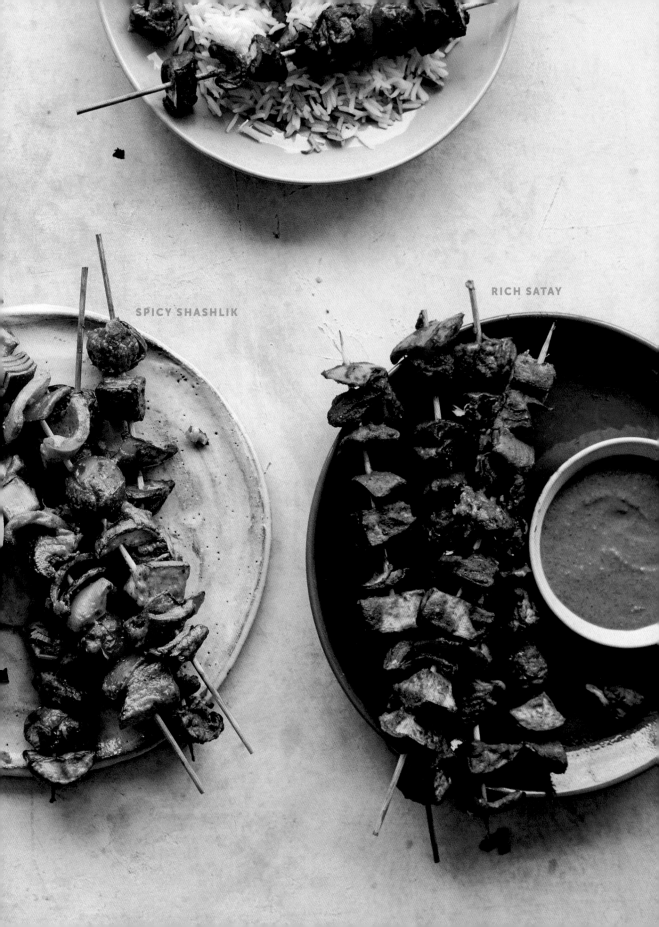

SPICY SHASHLIK

RICH SATAY

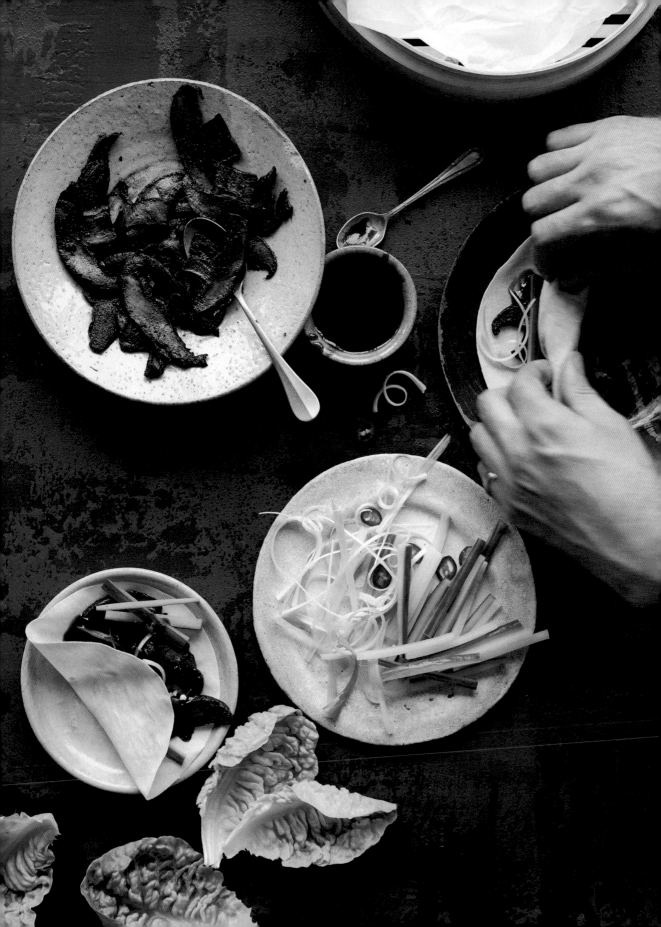

HOISIN PANCAKES

Everyone's favorite Chinese sharer—rich, salty mushrooms combine with the fresh green veggies and sweet hoisin sauce to create a starter that no one can refuse. This is delicious with Asian dishes like our Crispy Chili Tofu (see page 46) or Sticky Shiitake Mushrooms (see page 30). You can also replace the pancakes with gem lettuce leaves and simply wrap them into little healthy parcels.

SERVES 2 AS A STARTER

2 tsp vegetable oil
10 oz mushrooms (portobello, if possible)
2 tbsp soy sauce
1 tsp five-spice powder
1 tbsp rice vinegar
2 tsp toasted sesame oil
1 tsp sugar
½ cucumber
3 scallions
5 tbsp hoisin sauce
8 Chinese pancakes

Small frying pan over medium heat

Put the oil into the pan | Roughly slice the mushrooms, add them to the pan, and cook for 10 minutes until their juices have cooked off | Add the soy sauce, five-spice, rice vinegar, sesame oil, and sugar | Continue to cook, stirring continously until any additional sauce has mostly evaporated and the mushrooms are beautifully cooked and glazed

Meanwhile, halve the cucumber and remove the watery core with a spoon, then finely slice into 2-inch matchsticks | Trim the top and bottom of the scallions and cut them into matchsticks | Put the cucumber and scallions on a small plate and pour the hoisin sauce into a small dish

Heat the pancakes following the instructions on the packet

When the mushrooms are ready, transfer them to a plate and serve them alongside their accompaniments | To assemble the pancakes, simply take a little of each ingredient and wrap them up into delicious pancake rolls

FRENCH ONION SOUP

A French classic presented in near-classic form. This is one for those long winter nights when you need something soothing and warming, great as a starter or served with chunky bread (perhaps spread with our Garlic & Herb Cashew Cheese on page 210) as a hearty meal for two. Be patient with the onions and you'll be rewarded with incredible flavor.

SERVES 2–4

1¾ oz dried porcini mushrooms
3 cups boiling water
3 tbsp olive oil
6 large onions (about 1 lb 10 oz)
6 garlic cloves
1 tsp brown sugar
2 tbsp dry sherry or port
½ tsp balsamic vinegar
½ lemon
½ tsp sea salt
¼ tsp black pepper
chunky bread, to serve, optional

Large saucepan over medium heat

Put the mushrooms in a small bowl and cover with the boiling water

Pour the oil into the pan | Peel and finely slice the onions and add them to the pan | Peel and finely chop the garlic and add to the pan with 2 tablespoons of water | Stir everything together, reduce the heat to low, cover and cook very gently for 40 minutes, stirring every couple of minutes, until the onions turn a deep caramel color | Add a tablespoon of water every now and again to prevent the onions from sticking | After 40 minutes, add the sugar and stir

Strain the soaking liquid from the mushrooms into a bowl, squeezing out as much liquid as possible (keep the mushrooms for making a risotto or something else) | Pour the soaking liquid over the onions, add the sherry and balsamic vinegar, stir everything together, and bring to a boil | Immediately reduce the heat to low and simmer gently for 10 minutes

Squeeze in the juice from the lemon, catching any seeds in your other hand | Season with salt and pepper, spoon into bowls, and serve on its own or with chunky bread, if using, to mop up the soup

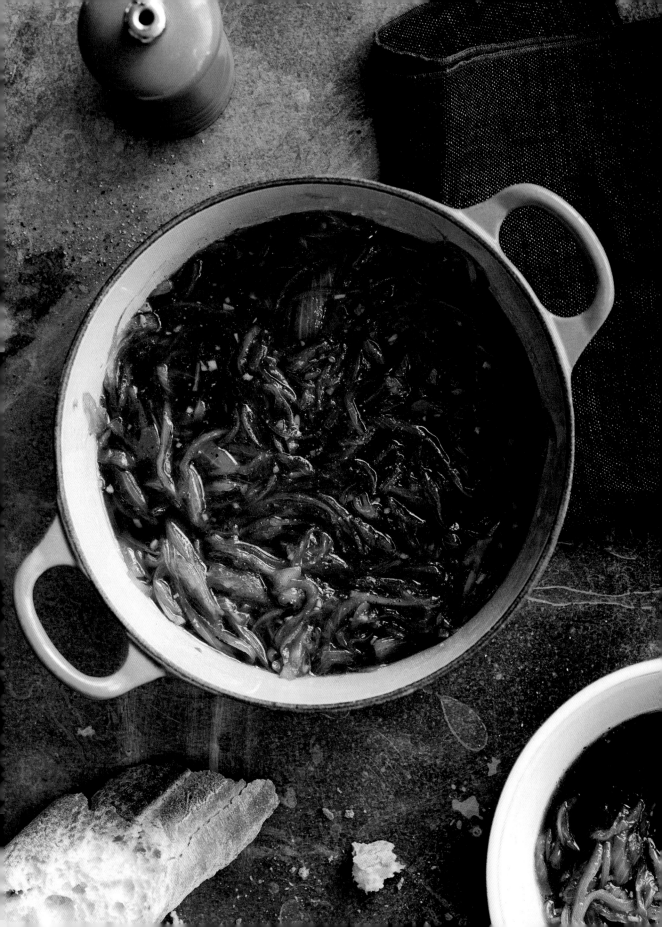

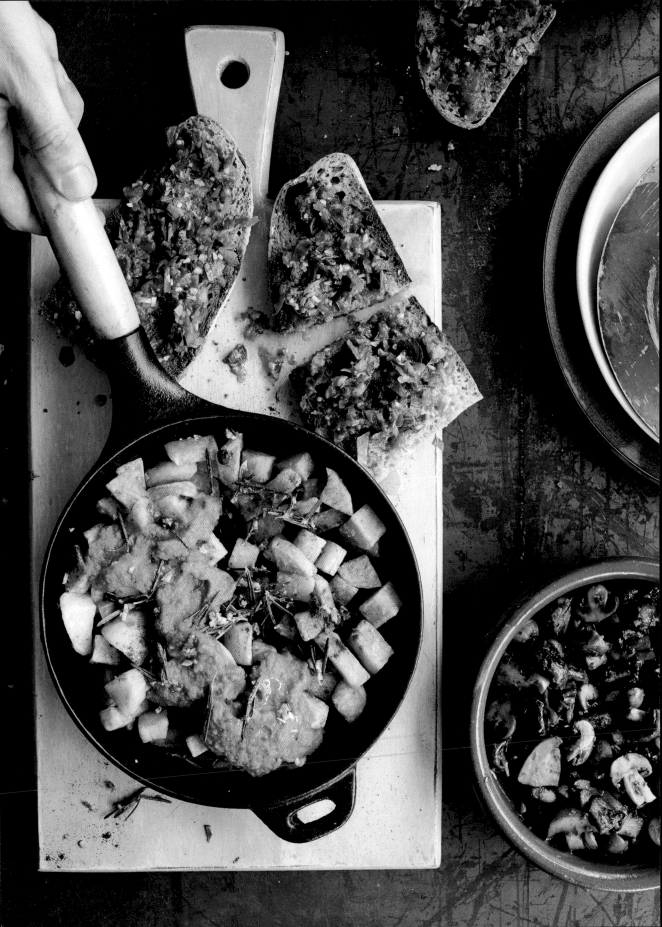

SPANISH TAPAS

Look no further for a Mediterranean feast! Any or all of these dishes would be great accompaniments to Pettigrew's Paella (see page 114), served alongside Proper Spanish Aioli (see page 192), Olive Tapenade (see page 192), and a small bowl of olives. Or why not try them as party canapés (if you can get past the garlic flavors!). And they would match perfectly with red wine.

JANE'S PAN CON TOMATE

Imagine an effortlessly simple Spanish bruschetta that's ready in minutes yet feels exotic. This one is a favorite of Henry's mum, Jane, and her well-honed Spanish palate.

MAKES 8 SLICES

Toaster or broiler | Coarse grater

3 tomatoes
3 garlic cloves
small handful fresh parsley
¼ cup olive oil
2 tbsp white wine vinegar or sherry vinegar
sugar, to season, optional
8 slices good-quality bread
salt and black pepper

Grate the tomatoes into a bowl | Peel the garlic and finely chop along with the parsley, then add to the bowl | Add the olive oil and vinegar and stir everything well | Taste and add salt, pepper, and even a little bit of sugar, if using, to taste

Slice the bread into ¾-inch-thick slices and toast or broil until lightly browned | Spread the tomato dressing all over the toast with a knife or the back of a spoon, rubbing the mixture into the bread, and serve

GARLIC MUSHROOMS

These are incredibly easy to cook and so, so tasty. Feel free
to use less garlic if you prefer, as this one's pretty punchy!

SERVES 4

11 oz cremini mushrooms
5 tbsp olive oil
½ fresh red chili
4 garlic cloves
½ cup dry white wine
½ lemon
salt

Large frying pan on a medium heat

Trim the mushrooms and cut them in half | Add the oil to the large
frying pan

Rip the stem from the chili, cut it in half lengthwise, and remove the
seeds, if you prefer a milder flavor, then finely chop and add to the pan |
Peel and finely chop the garlic, add it to the pan, and cook for 1 minute
before adding the sliced mushrooms | Fry for 3 minutes, stirring occasionally

Pour in the wine, turn up the heat to high, and cook for another 5 minutes,
stirring frequently, until the wine has reduced down to just a tablespoon
or so | Squeeze the lemon juice into the pan, catching any seeds in your
other hand | Cook for 1 more minute | Season to taste with salt and
more lemon, if desired

PATATAS BRAVAS

A staple in any good tapas restaurant, this is like the French fry's stronger, sexier Spanish cousin. The sauce is insane, the potatoes are perfectly cooked, the result is simple excellence. Feel free to use dried herbs if you don't have the fresh ones handy.

SERVES 2

4 potatoes
6 tbsp olive oil
1 onion
8 garlic cloves
4 fresh red chilies
½ carrot
1 tbsp fresh thyme leaves
1 can (14.5 oz) chopped tomatoes
1 tbsp white wine vinegar
3 sprigs fresh rosemary
1 tsp paprika
salt and black pepper

Large saucepan over medium heat | Medium frying pan over low heat | Large frying pan | Cover a plate with paper towels | Blender

Peel the potatoes and chop them into bite-sized pieces | Bring a large saucepan of water to a boil and add some salt | Add the potatoes and cook for 8–10 minutes until softened, but not falling apart

Meanwhile, pour 1 tablespoon of the olive oil into the medium frying pan | Peel and finely chop the onion and 3 of the garlic cloves and add them to the pan | Rip the stems from the chilies, cut them in half lengthwise, and remove the seeds if you prefer a milder sauce, then finely chop and add to the pan | Trim the carrot, finely chop, and add to the pan with the thyme leaves | Cook everything for 5–7 minutes, until the onion and carrot have softened

Add the chopped tomatoes to the pan along with the vinegar and salt and pepper to taste | Let the liquid come to a boil, then turn down the heat and simmer for 10 minutes

While the sauce is cooking, set the large frying pan over medium-high heat and pour in the remaining 5 tablespoons of olive oil, or enough to coat the bottom of the pan | Carefully add the softened potatoes and fry for about 10 minutes, turning them regularly, until golden and really crispy (the crispier the better)

Peel and finely chop the remaining garlic and add to the pan with the potatoes | Remove the rosemary leaves by running your thumb and forefinger from the top to the base of the stems (the leaves should easily come away), then finely chop and add to the pan | When they are ready, transfer to the paper towels and sprinkle with the paprika and a little salt; they should be lightly browned and crispy on the outside

Tip the tomato sauce into a blender and whizz to a smooth paste | Give it a taste before serving and adjust the flavor if you like, adding more salt or pepper as you see fit | Put the potatoes on a plate, pour the sauce over the top, and serve

PERI PERI HASSELBACK POTATOES

Halfway between a baked potato and a French fry, this quirky way to serve potatoes looks impressive but is simple to prepare. This goes great with a Big BOSH! Burger (see page 119) or as a side for a BBQ.

SERVES 4

4 large white potatoes
¼ cup olive oil, plus extra for drizzling
6 tbsp nondairy yogurt
paprika, to sprinkle
garlic powder, to sprinkle
1 tbsp hot sauce
1 tbsp chopped chives, to serve
sea salt

FOR THE PERI PERI SPICE RUB
1½ tsp paprika
1½ tsp onion powder
1 tsp garlic powder
1 tsp dried oregano
1 tsp ground ginger
½ tsp cayenne pepper
½ tsp salt

Preheat oven to 350°F

Place one of the potatoes on a cutting board and lay a wooden spoon on either side (these will provide a stopping point so that you don't cut all the way through your potatoes) | Take a sharp knife and carefully cut very thin slices crosswise along the full length of the potato, stopping when the knife hits the spoon handles | Repeat until all the potatoes have been "hasselbacked"

Cut 4 rectangles of foil large enough to cover each potato | Put one potato in the center of each and pull the sides up to form little nests | Drizzle 1 tablespoon olive oil over each potato, making sure the oil gets in between all the slices

Measure the spices for the spice rub into a small bowl and stir to combine | Use a teaspoon to sprinkle equal amounts of the spice rub over, and in between the slices of, each potato | Wrap the potatoes up in the foil ensuring there are no gaps | Place on a baking sheet, put the pan in the oven, and bake the potatoes for 45 minutes | Take the pan out of the oven and set it down on a heatproof mat | Turn the oven up to 425°F

Carefully open the parcels and flatten down the foil around the potatoes, being careful not to burn your fingers | Use the tip of a knife to lightly prise open the slices | Drizzle a touch more olive oil and sprinkle a little more salt over the potatoes | Put the pan back in the oven with the foil nests unwrapped and bake for 20–30 minutes longer

Spoon the yogurt into a small dish and sprinkle with paprika and garlic powder | Spoon some hot sauce on top and swirl it into the yogurt | Take the potatoes out of the oven | Lift them out of the foil nests and transfer to plates | Spoon the spice oil that's gathered in the foil nests over the potatoes | Garnish with chopped chives and serve with the spiced yogurt

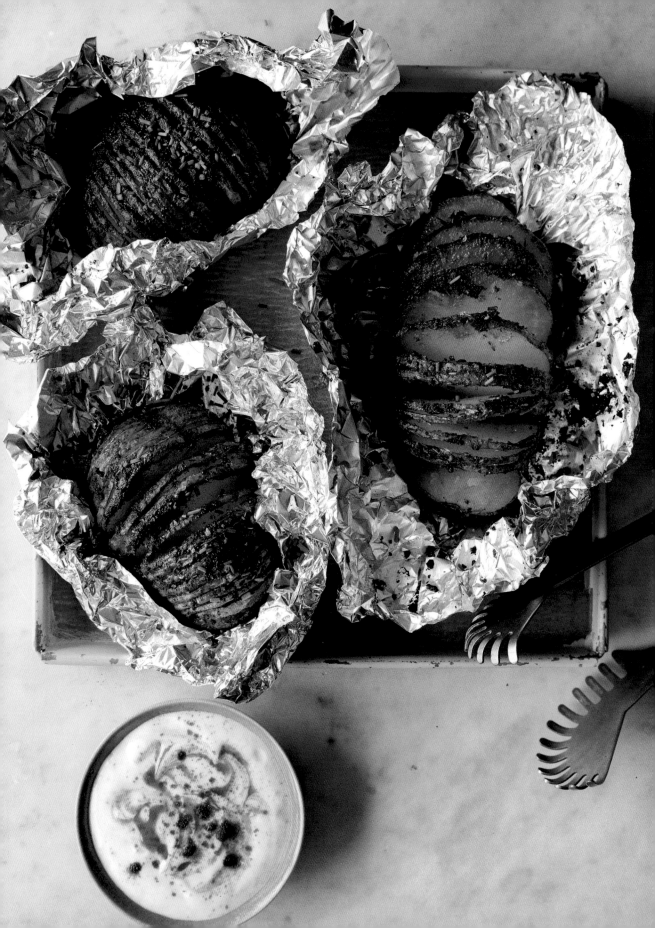

ALL THE SAUCES

Oh dips, how we love you. These quick-to-make, guaranteed-to-please dips add another level of flavor to any meal in this book and impress any of your dinner guests. They're perfect party fodder: try serving a selection with fries, bread, and sides for a buffet to rule them all. Or they are all delicious served with salads, pizzas, chips, crudités, you name it! See the whole selection in their rainbow of colors on page 196.

OLIVE TAPENADE

MAKES ABOUT 1¼ CUPS

Food processor or stick blender

7 oz black olives, such as Kalamata, preferably pitted
2 garlic cloves
3 tbsp capers
¾ cup fresh parsley, optional
½ lemon
5 tbsp olive oil

Remove the pits from the olives if they are not already pitted | Peel and crush the garlic into the food processor (or into a bowl if you're using a stick blender) and add the olives, capers, and parsley, if using | Squeeze in the juice from the lemon, catching any seeds in your other hand | Whizz to a rough purée

Pour in the olive oil bit by bit and give it a couple more pulses until very well combined, but still retaining some texture | Transfer to a serving bowl

PROPER SPANISH AIOLI

MAKES ⅓ CUP

Pestle and mortar (or use a small bowl and a wooden spoon)

5 garlic cloves
1 tsp sea salt
½ lemon
½ cup olive oil

Peel and thinly slice the garlic and put it in the mortar (or bowl) with the sea salt | Squeeze in the lemon juice, catching any seeds with your other hand | Bash to a fine pulp using the pestle (or wooden spoon) | Add a teaspoon of the oil and mash thoroughly into the garlic pulp, ensuring it is well mixed in | Repeat until all the oil is used up, making sure you only add a teaspoon of oil at a time and that each time the oil is fully incorporated before continuing, otherwise the mixture will split

RICH SATAY SAUCE

MAKES ¾ CUP

2 limes
1 fresh red chili
1 garlic clove
¾-inch piece fresh ginger
generous ½ cup good-quality crunchy
    peanut butter
⅔ cup fresh cilantro
1 tbsp soy sauce

Food processor or stick blender

Finely zest the limes, then cut them in half and squeeze out the juice, catching any seeds in your other hand | Rip the stem from the chili into the food processor or bowl and remove the seeds, if you prefer a milder sauce | Peel the garlic | Peel the ginger by scraping off the skin with a spoon

Add all the ingredients to the food processor or a bowl and blend until smooth | Test the consistency, adding 1–2 tablespoons water to get the sauce as runny as you like | Taste and season with more lime juice or soy sauce if necessary

BABA GANOUSH

MAKES ABOUT 1⅓ CUPS

2 medium eggplants (about 1 lb)
2 small garlic cloves
1 lemon
2 tbsp tahini
3 tbsp olive oil
1 tsp cumin seeds
½ tsp smoked paprika
½ tsp salt
any combination of fresh chopped
    parsley, chili flakes, and/or harissa
    paste, to serve, optional

Preheat oven to 465°F | Line a baking sheet | Food processor or stick blender

Pierce the skin of the eggplants a few times with a fork | Put onto the lined baking sheet and place on the highest rack in the oven | Cook for 20–25 minutes, turning once or twice, until the skin is blackened all over | Remove to a bowl and leave to cool

Meanwhile, peel the garlic and put it in the food processor (or a bowl) | Cut the lemon in half and squeeze in the juice, catching any seeds in your other hand | Add the tahini, olive oil, cumin, paprika, and salt

Cut the eggplant in half and use a large spoon to scoop out the flesh (or peel off the charred skin with your fingers) | Transfer the eggplant flesh to the food processor (or bowl) along with a few pieces of the charred skin to add flavor | Whizz until smooth

Taste and add a little more lemon juice or salt, if needed | Garnish with a few toppings, if using, such as the chopped parsley leaves, chili flakes, and/or harissa

AMAZING CHILI SAUCE

MAKES 1 CUP

2 red bell peppers
5 fresh red chilies
3 garlic cloves
7 tbsp white wine vinegar
¼ cup sugar
1 tbsp cornstarch
2 tsp water
1 lime
½ tsp salt

Stand blender or stick blender | Small pan over high heat

Cut the bell peppers in half and cut out the stems and seeds | Rip the stems from the chilies, cut them in half lengthwise, and remove the seeds | Peel the garlic cloves | Add to the blender or a bowl along with the vinegar and sugar and blend until completely smooth

Pour into the hot pan, bring to a boil, then lower the heat to medium and simmer for 5 minutes

Put the cornstarch in a mug with the water | Stir until the flour has dissolved and there are no lumps | Pour into the pan and continue to simmer, stirring continuously, for 2 minutes

Cut the lime in half and squeeze in the juice, catching any seeds in your other hand | Season with the salt | Remove from the heat and leave to cool

ULTIMATE GUACAMOLE

MAKES A SCANT 2 CUPS

1 fresh red chili
¼ red onion
12 cherry tomatoes
2 ripe avocados
15 sprigs fresh cilantro
1½ limes
1 tsp salt
1 tsp garlic powder
1½ tbsp olive oil

Rip the stem from the chili, cut it in half lengthwise, and remove the seeds, if you prefer a milder flavor, then finely chop | Peel and finely chop the onion and cherry tomatoes | Put the chopped vegetables into a bowl | Halve and carefully pit the avocados by tapping the pits firmly with the heel of a knife so that it lodges in the pits, then twist and remove the pits | Scoop the flesh into the bowl | Use the back of a fork or a potato masher to roughly mash the avocados, making sure you keep some lumps for texture

Discard any large stems from the cilantro and finely chop the leaves | Add to the bowl | Cut the limes in half and squeeze over the juice, catching any seeds in your other hand | Add the salt, garlic powder, and olive oil and stir everything together with a wooden spoon | Taste and adjust the seasoning as desired

BANGIN' SALSA

MAKES A GENEROUS 1 CUP

2 fresh red chilies
1 red or yellow bell pepper
2 scallions
3 tomatoes
¼ cucumber
1 lime
2 tbsp red wine vinegar
handful fresh basil
salt and black pepper

Rip the stems from the chilies, cut them in half lengthwise, and remove the seeds, if you prefer a milder flavor, then finely chop | Cut the bell pepper in half and cut out the stem and seeds | Trim and finely slice the scallions | Finely dice the tomatoes | Cut the cucumber in half lengthwise and scrape out the watery middle with a teaspoon, then finely dice | Put everything in a bowl

Zest the lime, cut it in half, and squeeze the juice into the bowl, catching any seeds in your other hand | Add the red wine vinegar and tear the basil leaves into the bowl | Season with salt and pepper to taste

FIERY CHILI PESTO

MAKES ABOUT 1 CUP

1 garlic clove
1 fresh red chili
6 oz roasted red peppers, from a jar
2 tbsp pine nuts
1¼ cups fresh basil leaves
½ tsp salt
½ lemon
1 tbsp olive oil
1 tbsp nutritional yeast, optional
1 tsp agave nectar
2 tsp tomato paste

Food processor

Peel the garlic | Rip the stem from the chili, cut it in half lengthwise, and remove the seeds if you prefer a milder pesto | Add both to the food processor | Add the roasted red peppers, pine nuts, basil, and salt | Squeeze in the juice of the lemon, catching any seeds with your other hand | Add the olive oil, nutritional yeast, if using, agave nectar, and tomato paste

Whizz together until everything is ground down to a creamy pesto, still with a bit of texture

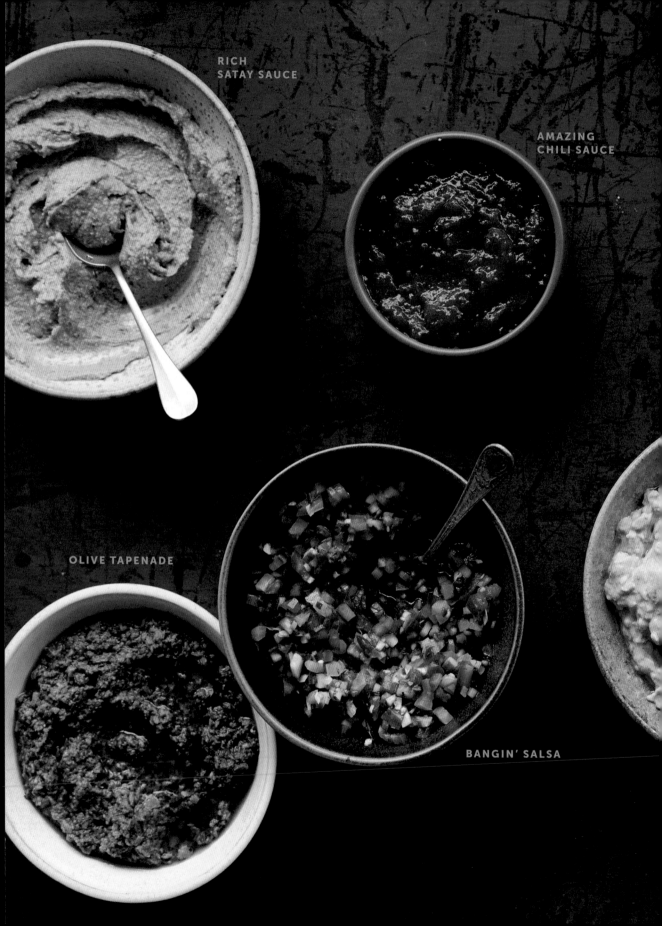

RICH
SATAY SAUCE

AMAZING
CHILI SAUCE

OLIVE TAPENADE

BANGIN' SALSA

ULTIMATE
GUACAMOLE

FIERY
CHILI PESTO

BABA GANOUSH

PROPER
SPANISH AIOLI

ALL THE HUMMUS

Simple, tasty, and universally loved, the wonderful hummus is a must in any discerning cook's repertoire. We like to freestyle with ours and create different flavors, each one a slightly remixed version of the original. So rather than give you one dish, here are eight ideas for how you could pay your own respects to the granddaddy of dips, the lifelong partner of falafel. Check out the photos overleaf to see the mouthwatering options.

Hummus is effortless to make—5 minutes with a blender and you are done. Our classic recipe is used in our Mezze Cake (see page 98), Middle East Pizza (see page 108), and would go well with pretty much any dish in this book.

ROASTED GARLIC HUMMUS

MAKES ABOUT 1¼ CUPS

1 large garlic bulb (5–10 cloves)
1 can (15 oz) chickpeas
1 tbsp tahini
1 tsp salt
2 tbsp lemon juice
2 tbsp olive oil
2 tbsp water
½ oz fresh chives

Preheat oven to 320°F | Food processor

Put the garlic bulb on a baking sheet, put the pan in the oven, and roast for 30 minutes | Remove and leave to cool, then peel | Drain the chickpeas | Put the roasted garlic, chickpeas, tahini, salt, lemon juice, oil, and water into the food processor and whizz to a smooth paste | Finely chop the chives and stir them in at the end

SUN-DRIED TOMATO HUMMUS

MAKES ABOUT 1¼ CUPS

1 can (15 oz) chickpeas
1 garlic clove
5 sun-dried tomatoes
½ tsp dried oregano
¼ tsp sea salt
2 tbsp lemon juice
1 tbsp sun-dried tomato oil from the jar

Food processor

Drain the chickpeas | Peel the garlic | Put all the ingredients into the food processor | Whizz to a smooth paste and serve

OLIVE TAPENADE HUMMUS

MAKES ABOUT 1¼ cups

1 can (15 oz) chickpeas
1 garlic clove
⅓ cup pitted Kalamata olives
1 roasted red pepper from a jar
1¼ cups fresh parsley leaves
¼ tsp sea salt
2 tbsp lemon juice
2 tbsp olive oil

Food processor

Drain the chickpeas | Peel the garlic | Put all the ingredients into the food processor | Whizz to a smooth paste and serve

BURRITO HUMMUS

MAKES ABOUT 1¼ CUPS

1 can (15 oz) black beans
⅔ cup fresh cilantro leaves
1 tsp ground cumin
½ tsp salt
¼ tsp black pepper
2 tbsp lime juice
2 tsp chipotle sauce

Food processor

Drain the black beans | Put all the ingredients into the food processor | Whizz to a smooth paste and serve

CLASSIC HUMMUS

MAKES ABOUT 1¼ CUPS

1 can (15 oz) chickpeas
2 small garlic cloves
2 tbsp tahini
¾ tsp salt
¼ cup water
2½ tbsp lemon juice
2 tbsp olive oil

Food processor

Drain the chickpeas | Peel the garlic | Put all the ingredients into the food processor | Whizz to a smooth paste and serve

PESTO HUMMUS

MAKES ABOUT 1¼ CUPS

1 can (15 oz) chickpeas
1 garlic clove
¾ cup fresh basil leaves
2 tbsp tahini
1 tbsp nutritional yeast
½ tsp salt
3 tbsp water
2½ tbsp lemon juice
2 tbsp olive oil

Food processor

Drain the chickpeas | Peel the garlic | Put all the ingredients into the food processor | Whizz to a smooth paste and serve

GUACUMMUS

MAKES ABOUT 1¼ CUPS

1¼ cups canned chickpeas
1 avocado
1 tbsp fresh cilantro leaves
¾ tsp salt
½ tsp chili flakes
2 tbsp lime juice
2 tbsp olive oil
2 tbsp water

Food processor

Drain the chickpeas | Halve and carefully pit the avocado by tapping the pit firmly with the heel of a knife so that it lodges in the pit, then twist and remove the pit | Scoop the flesh into the food processor and add the rest of the ingredients | Whizz to a smooth paste and serve

SATAY HUMMUS

MAKES ABOUT 1¼ CUPS

1 can (15 oz) chickpeas
3 tbsp smooth peanut butter
1 tsp smoked paprika
1 tsp chili flakes
¼ tsp sea salt
2 tbsp unsweetened plant-based milk
2 tbsp water
1 tbsp olive oil
1 tbsp lime juice
1 tsp soy sauce

Food processor

Drain the chickpeas | Put all the ingredients into the food processor | Whizz to a smooth paste and serve

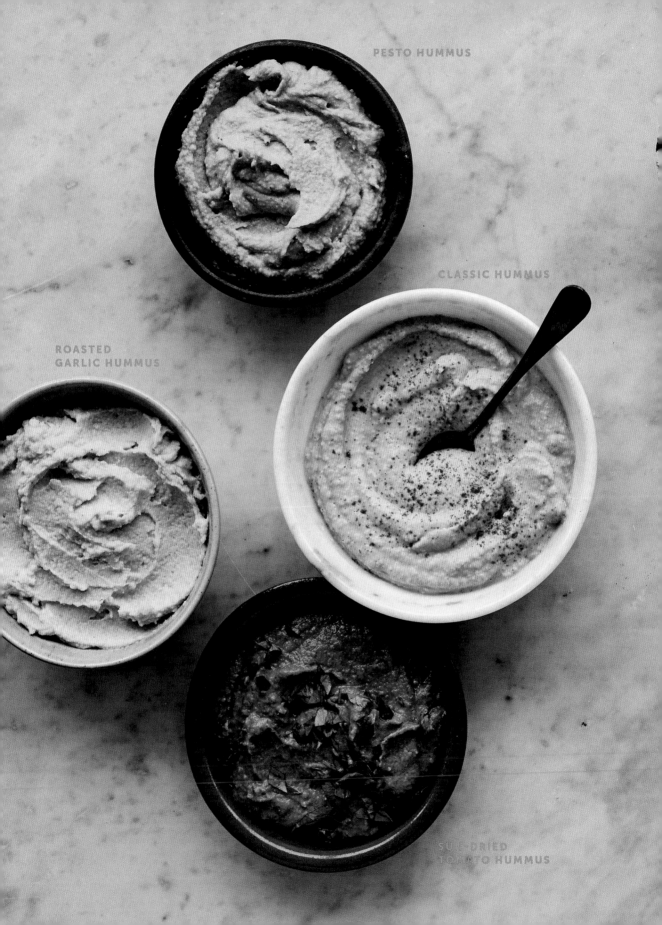

PESTO HUMMUS

CLASSIC HUMMUS

ROASTED
GARLIC HUMMUS

SUN-DRIED
TOMATO HUMMUS

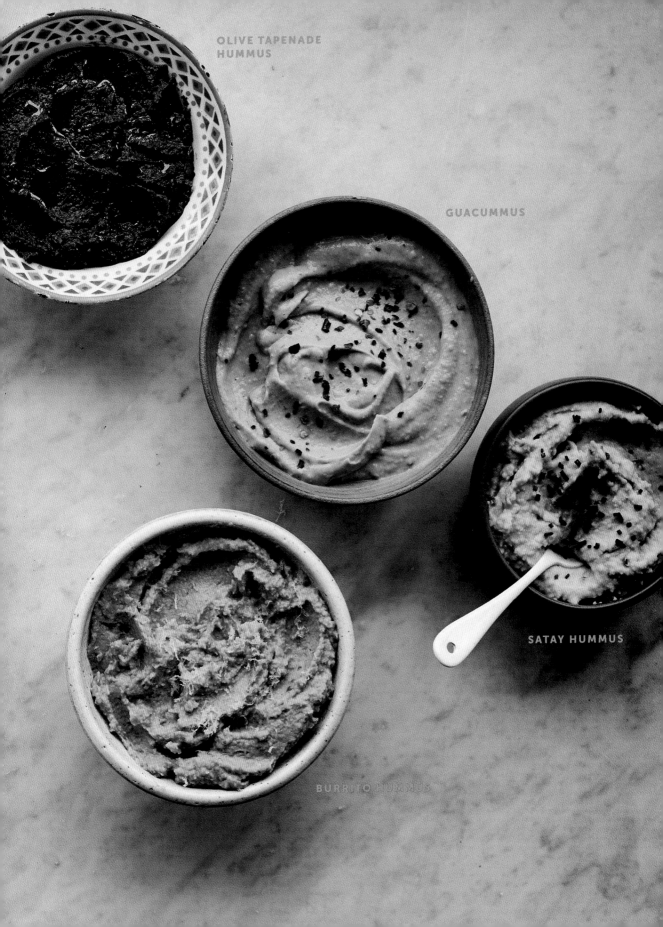

OLIVE TAPENADE
HUMMUS

GUACUMMUS

SATAY HUMMUS

BURRITO HUMMUS

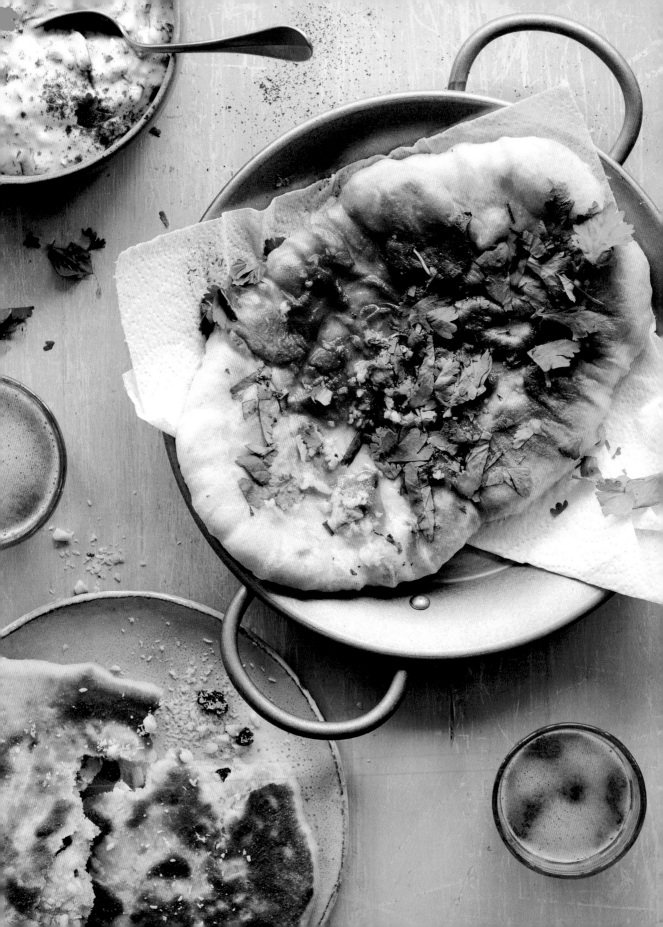

FLUFFY NAAN BREAD & RAITA

Indian meals are such fun and for us it's so much more satisfying to have a fluffy naan bread to complement your core curries. These breads and accompanying raita dip are quick to prepare and will ensure a home-cooked feast that transcends any takeout. The naans are easy enough; just give them a bit of time to rise. Trust us, it's worth it.

BASIC NAAN BREAD

MAKES 4 LARGE NAAN BREADS

FOR THE BASIC NAAN DOUGH
1 envelope (¼ oz) active dry yeast
¾ cup + 3 tbsp warm water
2 tbsp sugar
6 tbsp unsweetened plant-based milk
2 tsp salt
3 cups bread flour, plus extra for dusting
vegetable oil

Large mixing bowl | Stand mixer fitted with the dough hook, or dust a clean work surface liberally with flour | Large frying pan | Rolling pin or a clean, dry wine bottle | Pastry brush

Put the yeast and warm water into the mixing bowl and stir to combine | Set aside for 10–15 minutes until the mixture has started to froth

Once the yeast has activated, add the sugar, plant-based milk, salt, and flour | Stir with a wooden spoon and bring it together to form a soft and sticky dough | Transfer the dough to the stand mixer, if using, and knead for 6 minutes; otherwise tip it onto the floured work surface, dust your hands with more flour, and knead for 10–12 minutes by pushing the back half of the dough away with the heel of one hand, folding it back over the dough, giving it a quarter turn and repeating

Clean and dry the mixing bowl and grease the inside with a little vegetable oil | Place the dough in the bowl, cover it loosely with plastic wrap or a plastic bag, and leave it in a warm spot for 60–90 minutes, or until it's doubled in size

Once the dough has doubled in size, knock out the air by punching it in the bowl and then knead for another 1–2 minutes | Dust the work surface with at least 6 tablespoons of flour | Turn out the dough and coat it in the flour so that it's no longer sticky | Roll the dough into a ball and use a sharp knife to divide it in half and then half again, so that you have 4 equal balls of dough weighing about 6 oz each | Roll each ball in flour again to prevent sticking

Dust the rolling pin or wine bottle with more flour and roll out the balls of dough to form rough teardrop shapes

Pour 1 tablespoon vegetable oil into the large frying pan and set it over medium heat

One by one, fry the naans for 5 minutes, turning them over halfway through, until golden and slightly charred on both sides (if they puff up during cooking, flatten them down firmly with a spatula to ensure they cook through) | Remove the naans from the pan

GARLIC NAAN BREAD

The classic. Garlicky and a little oily, this is so moreish it will guarantee you are full after your meal. You'll also feel like a master chef creating a naan from scratch.

MAKES 4 LARGE NAAN BREADS

Basic Naan dough (see page 203)
¼ cup olive oil
5 garlic cloves
small handful fresh cilantro leaves, to serve
salt

Large mixing bowl | Stand mixer fitted with the dough hook, or dust a clean work surface liberally with flour | Small saucepan | Large frying pan | Rolling pin or a clean, dry wine bottle | Pastry brush

Make the naan dough following the instructions for Basic Naan Bread (see page 203)

While the dough is rising, pour the olive oil into the small saucepan | Peel and crush the garlic cloves into the pan | Set the pan over medium heat and cook the garlic until it turns just slightly golden, about 1–2 minutes (it will cook a bit more once it's off the burner, so make sure you don't overcook it) | Sprinkle with a small pinch of salt and set aside

Fry the naans for 5 minutes, turning them over halfway through, until golden and slightly charred on both sides (if they puff up during cooking, flatten them down firmly with a spatula to ensure they cook through) | Remove them from the pan and, while they're still hot, liberally brush each naan on both sides with the garlic oil | Scatter with some fresh cilantro leaves and serve immediately

JANE'S MINT RAITA

Henry's mum taught him this incredibly simple dish at a young age. It's basically just yogurt, mint, and veg, but the addition of lemon gives it a real zing. Feel free to experiment with different veg combinations; it can be made with fresh mint, but we find the tart mint sauce contrasts well with the sugar.

SERVES 2–4

scant 1 cup nondairy yogurt
½ onion
½ tomato, or about 6 cherry tomatoes
¼ cucumber
½ tsp sugar
½ tsp salt
2 tsp mint sauce
pinch of cayenne pepper, plus a little extra to serve
½ lemon

Put the yogurt into a bowl | Peel and finely chop the onion and add it to the bowl | Finely chop the tomato and cucumber and add them to the bowl with the sugar, salt, mint sauce, and cayenne pepper | Squeeze in the juice of the lemon, catching any seeds in your other hand | Taste and adjust the seasoning if necessary | Sprinkle over a little more cayenne pepper to serve for a splash of color

PESHWARI NAAN BREAD

Peshwari naans are so sweet and delicious it's almost like eating a dessert. But a good one improves any savory dish it's eaten with, the little crumbly bits of coconut falling out adding an extra topping to your curry. They are surprisingly easy to make—and totally worth it.

MAKES 4 LARGE NAAN BREADS

Basic Naan dough (see page 203)
3 oz blanched almonds
3 tbsp raisins
2 tbsp superfine sugar
5 tbsp shredded coconut
3 tbsp vegetable oil

Large mixing bowl | Stand mixer fitted with the dough hook, or dust a clean work surface liberally with flour | Blender | Rolling pin or a clean, dry wine bottle | Large frying pan

Make the naan dough following the instructions for Basic Naan Bread (see page 203), up to where the dough is divided into 4 pieces

Put the almonds, raisins, sugar, and coconut into the blender and whizz for 1–2 minutes, until you have a coarse mixture

Flour the rolling pin or wine bottle and roll out one ball of dough to a rough round | Place a quarter of the filling mixture into the center of the round | Dust your hands with flour, lift up the edges of the dough with your fingers, and pinch them together in the center so that the filling is fully enclosed | Gently flatten the filled dough ball and roll it out into a rough teardrop shape | Repeat with the remaining balls of dough and filling

Pour the vegetable oil into the large frying pan and set it over medium heat | One by one, fry the naans for 5 minutes, turning them over halfway through, until golden and slightly charred on both sides (if they puff up during cooking, flatten them down firmly with a spatula to ensure they cook through) | Remove the naans from the pan and serve immediately

SPECIAL
FRIED RICE

PERFECTLY
BOILED RICE

ONION
FRIED RICE

RICE 3 WAYS

Humans have been thriving on rice for centuries. Here we'll show you an awesome way to cook it, taught to Henry by his father, that will ensure your rice is perfect every time. And what's even better than rice? Fried rice, obviously. We love it as a speedy dish to enjoy on its own or to jazz up any meal. You can also speed things up by using precooked rice, which is available in most supermarkets.

PERFECTLY BOILED RICE

This is a really neat way to ensure perfect rice every time. You could add a knob of peeled ginger, a slice of lemon, or a jasmine teabag for flavored rice. It's super simple. Just remember: double the quantity of water to rice, lid on, lowest heat, 12 minutes, BOSH! Works every time.

SERVES 1–2

½ mug basmati rice (about ½ cup)
1 mug boiling water (about 1 cup)
salt

Medium pan with a tight-fitting lid over high heat

Rinse the rice under cold running water | Drain and transfer to the pan | Add the freshly boiled water and a large pinch of salt | Put the lid on and bring to a boil | Give one stir with a spoon and immediately reduce the heat to the lowest setting | Put the lid back on and cook for 12 minutes | Don't touch the rice until the time is up

After the timer has gone off, take the pan off the heat

ONION FRIED RICE

This wonderful rice will add a little extra to any Indian curry. It's quick, simple, but delicious. Try alongside our Rogan BOSH! (see page 74), Creamy Korma (see page 71), and Garlic Naan (see page 204).

SERVES 1–2

1 small red onion
2-inch piece fresh ginger
2 tbsp vegetable oil
1 tbsp cumin seeds
2 tbsp soy sauce
½ tsp chili flakes, optional
Perfectly Boiled Rice (see page 207) or
    1½ cups store-bought precooked
    basmati rice

Large frying pan over medium heat

Peel and thinly slice the onion | Peel the ginger by scraping off the skin with a spoon and finely grate

Add the oil to the frying pan | Add the cumin seeds and fry for about 1 minute until they are a shade darker and aromatic | Add the grated ginger and fry for another minute

Add the red onion and continue to fry for 5–6 minutes, until the onion is softened | Add the soy sauce, chili flakes, if using, and the cooked rice | Combine everything together and serve immediately

SPECIAL FRIED RICE

This gorgeous fried rice is good enough to eat on its own, but would also work perfectly with any Thai or Chinese main course. It's also great for a quick feed when you get home after a late night!

SERVES 1–2

3 oz firm tofu
3 garlic cloves
2 scallions
1 small carrot
1 small red bell pepper
1½ tbsp vegetable oil
1 tbsp toasted sesame oil
⅓ cup green peas
⅓ cup corn
1 tsp ground turmeric
1 tsp curry powder
½ tsp black pepper
1 tbsp brown sugar
1 tbsp dairy-free butter or spread
Perfectly Boiled Rice (see page 207) or
    1½ cups store-bought precooked
    basmati rice
3 tbsp soy sauce
handful fresh cilantro, to serve
salt

Tofu press or 2 clean kitchen towels and a weight such as a heavy book | Saucepan | Wok or large frying pan over high heat

Press the tofu using a tofu press or place it between two clean kitchen towels, lay it on a plate, and put a weight on top | Leave for at least 30 minutes to drain any liquid and firm up before you start cooking

Peel and finely chop the garlic | Trim the roots of the scallions, roughly chop the green parts, and finely chop the white stems | Peel the carrot and chop it into ¼-inch dice | Cut the bell pepper in half and cut out the stem and seeds, then slice into ¼-inch dice

Pour the oils into the wok or frying pan | Add the carrot, bell pepper, garlic, and scallions, leaving aside some of the green parts to scatter over later | Stir-fry for 1 minute

Crumble in rough pieces of the tofu | Add the peas, corn, turmeric, curry powder, black pepper, and sugar | Stir-fry for another 6–8 minutes, until the vegetables are cooked through | Add the dairy-free butter, rice, and soy sauce and stir everything together | Season with salt to taste

Garnish with the cilantro leaves and the remaining chopped scallions and serve immediately

GARLIC & HERB CASHEW CHEESE

It's amazing how easy it is to make delicious, healthy cream cheese from mostly pantry ingredients. If we need a quick cheese to go in a pasta or on toast, this is our go-to recipe. Cashews are the magic ingredient here and you'll need a badboy blender to get the cheese nice and smooth.

MAKES 1¾ CUPS

11 oz cashews
4 tbsp water
1 tsp salt
2 tbsp coconut oil
1 tbsp nutritional yeast
1 lemon
1 garlic clove
small handful fresh parsley leaves
6–8 chives

Medium saucepan of water over high heat | Food processor or blender

Put the cashews in the pan of hot water and boil for 15 minutes until they are soft and have rehydrated (alternatively, you can soak them overnight in cold water) | Drain the nuts and tip them into a food processor or blender with 2 tbsp of the fresh water | Whizz for 60 seconds until you have a thick, smooth, creamy paste with no bits

Add the remaining 2 tbsp water, the salt, coconut oil, and nutritional yeast (you want a thick, gloopy consistency, so add more water if necessary) | Cut the lemon in half and squeeze in the juice, catching any seeds in your other hand | Peel the garlic and add it to the food processor or blender | Whizz for a few minutes until the mixture is very smooth, scraping down the sides with a spatula every now and then to make sure everything is mixed

Transfer the completely smooth mixture to a bowl | Finely chop the parsley and chives and stir them into the mixture with a spoon

Lay out a large piece of plastic wrap on a clean work surface and spoon the mixture into the middle | Fold over the plastic wrap and roll up the cheese into a log, squeezing out any air and tightening the ends of the plastic wrap as you go | Refrigerate for at least 2 hours to set fully

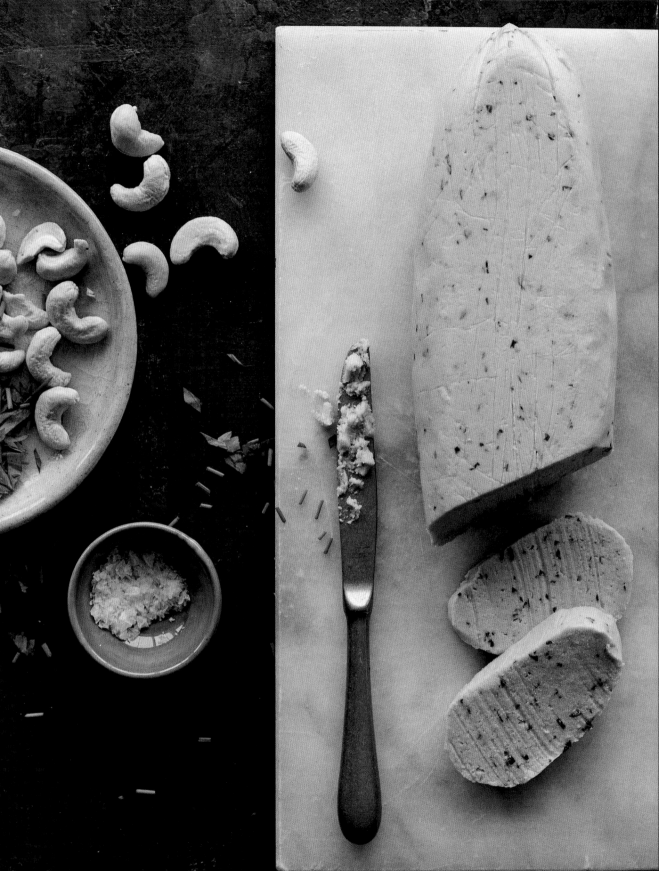

06

COCKTAILS

When you're in the mood
Reach for the cocktail shaker
And wow with these drinks

EASY ALMOND BAILEYS

You can make this quick version of Baileys in less than five minutes. It was inspired by our favorite bartenders, Susie and Tim, and it's the drink to cozy up in front of a movie with. Make a big batch and leave it in the fridge for up to a week; just give it a good shake before serving.

MAKES 2⅓ CUPS

Large pitcher | Shot measure | Tumblers

1⅔ cups unsweetened almond milk
¼ cup Jack Daniel's
3 tbsp freshly brewed espresso
3 tbsp agave syrup or maple syrup
1 tsp vanilla extract
ice, to serve, optional

Measure all the ingredients into a large pitcher and stir with a fork until mixed | Serve neat in tumblers over ice, if using

SALTED CARAMEL ESPRESSO MARTINI

This is a fantastic way to feel both sophisticated and a little bit excited. Just whack some caffeine in your drink to add instant liveliness to your evening. Espresso martinis are a go-to in the BOSH! household. Just make sure to be responsible—one or two of these beauties is plenty! Everyone who tries this goes "mmm" and a photo is guaranteed.

MAKES 2 MARTINI GLASSES

2 martini glasses | Cocktail shaker

8–10 ice cubes
5 tsp coffee liqueur (like Kahlúa)
3 tbsp + 1 tsp vodka
3 tbsp + 1 tsp brewed espresso
2 tsp caramel syrup
½ tsp salt
6 coffee beans, to serve

Put some ice in your empty martini glasses to cool them down | Fill the cocktail shaker with ice

Put the coffee liqueur, vodka, espresso, caramel syrup, and salt into the cocktail shaker, put the lid on, and shake vigorously to mix

Pour into the chilled glasses, decorate with the coffee beans, and serve

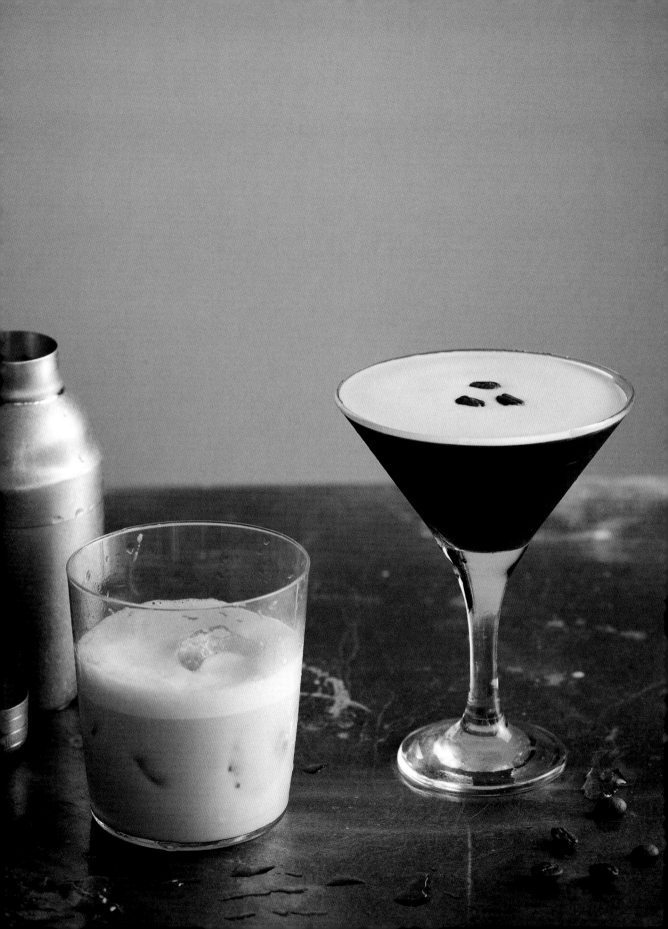

SMOOCHIES

If you're gonna be drinking, why not give yourself the gift of some nutrients at the same time? That's the inspiration behind our "Smoochies"—hooch smoothies. Why not create your own Smoochie bar at your next party and let your guests make their own? We call this pre-hab—getting your good deeds done in advance (of a boozy night, that is). Drink a few of these and you'll be merry but also glowing and full of antioxidants, vitamins, and goodness. You may still have a hangover, so don't drink too many!

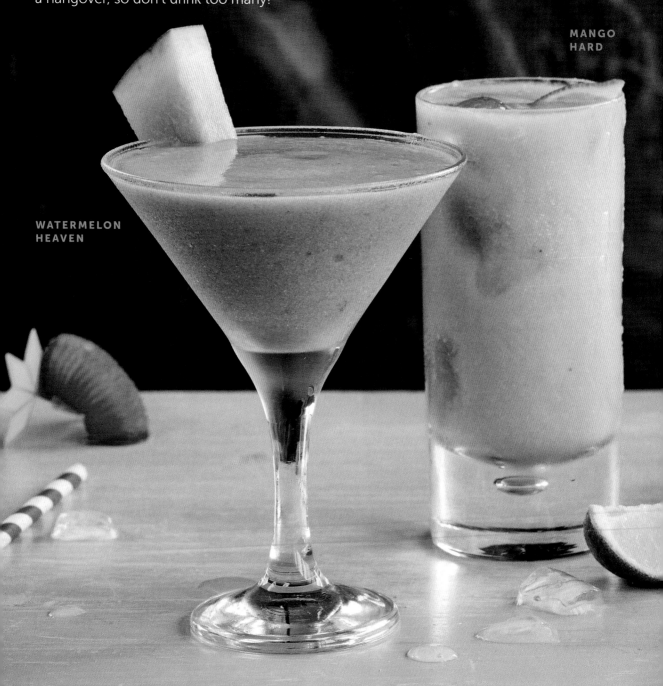

MANGO HARD

WATERMELON HEAVEN

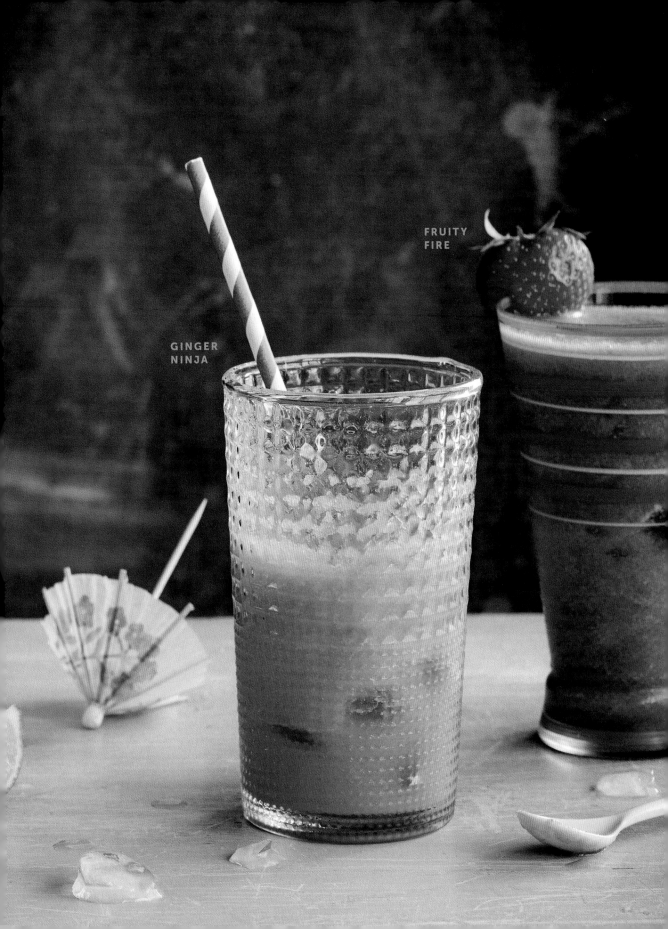

GINGER
NINJA

FRUITY
FIRE

WATERMELON HEAVEN

This is deliciously daiquiri-like, but filled with fruit and flavor
and just a touch of merry rum.

MAKES 4 MARTINI GLASSES | **Blender | 4 martini glasses | Paper straws, optional**

1 mango (about 8 oz)
5 oz strawberries
1 lime
6 oz frozen watermelon chunks
⅓ cup green grapes
1 slice fresh pineapple (about 3½ oz)
2 ice cubes, plus a little extra
½ cup spiced rum
fresh watermelon slices, to serve

Peel the mango and cut as much flesh from the pit as you can | Remove the hulls from the strawberries

Cut the lime in half and squeeze the juice into the blender, catching any seeds in your other hand, then add all the fruit and the ice cubes | Pour in the rum | Whizz it all up until it's like a thick, cold slushy | Add more ice if you need to make it thicker

Serve in martini glasses with slices of fresh watermelon on the side and paper straws, if using

GINGER NINJA

Ginger, carrots, orange and vodka—that's gotta be healthy,
right? It's also delicious. This really is a guilt-free party!

MAKES 4 GLASSES | **Blender | 4 highball glasses**

1-inch piece fresh ginger
10 oz carrots (3 medium)
1 orange
⅔ cup water
2 tbsp maple or agave syrup
⅔ cup vodka
½ lime
ice, to serve

Peel the ginger by scraping off the skin with a spoon | Trim the carrots | Peel the orange and remove the pith

Put the ginger, carrots, orange, water, syrup, and vodka into the blender | Squeeze in the lime juice, catching any seeds in your other hand, and whizz until completely smooth

Fill the glasses with ice, pour over the drink, and enjoy!

FRUITY FIRE

Fresh watermelon is a delicious, feel-good ingredient guaranteed to make you feel healthy and happy all at the same time. Add strawberries, banana, pineapple, and lime and you are in for a win! This is ready-made summer in a glass, and full of natural goodness.

MAKES 4 GLASSES

Blender | 4 highball glasses

4 oz fresh strawberries, plus 4 to serve
½ ripe banana (about 1¾ oz)
3½ oz fresh pineapple
8 oz fresh watermelon
   (without the rind)
1 lime
½ orange
⅔–¾ cup spiced rum
ice, to serve

Remove the hulls from the strawberries and peel the banana | Cut the skin off the pineapple and trim the top and bottom, then cut into chunks | Add all the fruit to the blender, squeezing in the lime and orange juice, catching any seeds in your other hand | Whizz until smooth | Add ⅔ cup of the rum, and add more to taste

Put some ice in your serving glasses | Pour in the boozy smoothie and garnish with a strawberry wedged onto the side of each glass

MANGO HARD

We are big rum fans and the combination of mango, banana, and spiced rum is simply delicious. It'll transport you away to a beach in the Caribbean, if only for a moment. And the goodness in all the fruit has gotta be good in your body, right?

MAKES 4 GLASSES

Blender | 4 highball glasses

½ apple (about 3 oz)
1 orange (about 4 oz peeled weight)
½ banana (about 1¾ oz)
½ mango (about 4 oz)
1 cup (about 4 oz) ice cubes,
   plus extra to serve
½–⅔ cup spiced rum
1 lime, to serve

Peel and core the apple | Peel the orange and remove the pith | Peel the banana | Peel the mango and cut as much flesh as you can from the pit | Add all the fruit except the lime to the blender with the ice cubes and the spiced rum and whizz until smooth | Cut the lime into slices

Serve the smoochie with ice and the slices of fresh lime

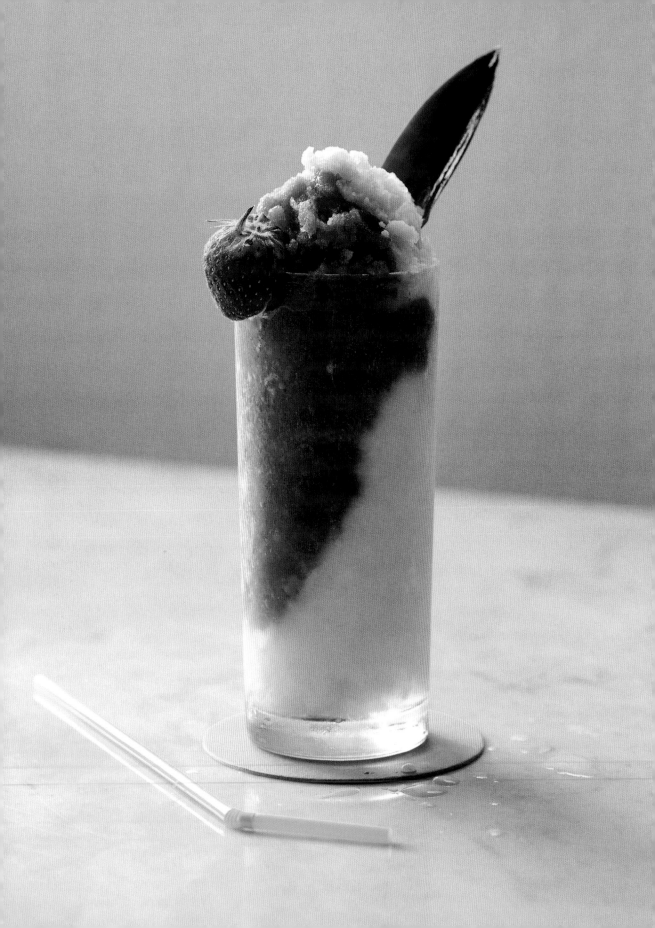

MIAMI VICE

Henry discovered this cocktail on a trip to the Bahamas and the flavors will take you straight there. It's an unbelievably tasty mix of strawberry daiquiri and piña colada—the perfect summer cocktail—and it's super impressive to behold. Get it really thick as it will melt as you drink it—you'll need a straw for this one!

MAKES TWO 16-OZ GLASSES

FOR SIMPLE SYRUP (WITH LEFTOVERS)
1 cup water
1 cup superfine sugar

FOR THE STRAWBERRY DAIQUIRI
9 oz strawberries
1 tbsp grenadine
¼ cup white rum
12–24 ice cubes

FOR THE PIÑA COLADA
3 tbsp coconut cream
3 tbsp pineapple juice
pineapple slice, optional
¼ cup white rum
12–24 ice cubes
2 strawberries, to decorate

Small saucepan over medium heat | Blender | Pitcher | Two 16-oz glasses | Straws (we recommend paper straws—they're better for the planet!)

To make a simple syrup, put the water and sugar into the saucepan and warm through for about 5 minutes, stirring continuously until all the sugar has dissolved | Remove from the heat and leave to cool | Keep any syrup you don't use in the fridge for another time

Next make the strawberry daiquiri | Remove the hulls from the strawberries and put the fruits into the blender with the grenadine, white rum, and 3 tbsp of the simple syrup you made earlier | Add 12 ice cubes and blend to a beautiful purée | If it's not so thick that it hardly moves, add more ice; you are looking for a thick, snow-like consistency | Once it's a very thick, smooth purée, pour it into a pitcher | Rinse out the blender

Now make the piña colada | Put the coconut cream, pineapple juice, 3 tbsp simple syrup, pineapple slice, if using, and white rum into the blender | Add 12 ice cubes and blend, aiming for a thick, stiff-peak consistency as before | Add more ice if you need to

Put a large wooden or metal serving spoon in the middle of one of the glasses | Pour both cocktail mixtures into the glass at the same time, one on either side of the spoon (you may need a friend to help you with this) | Pour all the way to the top, leaving a nice icy bump way above the top of the glass | Remove the spoon | Repeat with the second glass | Top your cocktails with fresh strawberries, pop in straws, and enjoy your culinary trip to the Bahamas!

MOJITOS

Rum. Lime. Mint. Spice. A quartet of wins makes these mojitos amazing. Perfect on a summer's day, they are fresh, crispy, and sweet, but with exotic, spicy flavors that are perfect with Asian dishes. Mojitos are usually made with a muddler to squash the lime, but the bottom of a rolling pin or a spoon will work just fine.

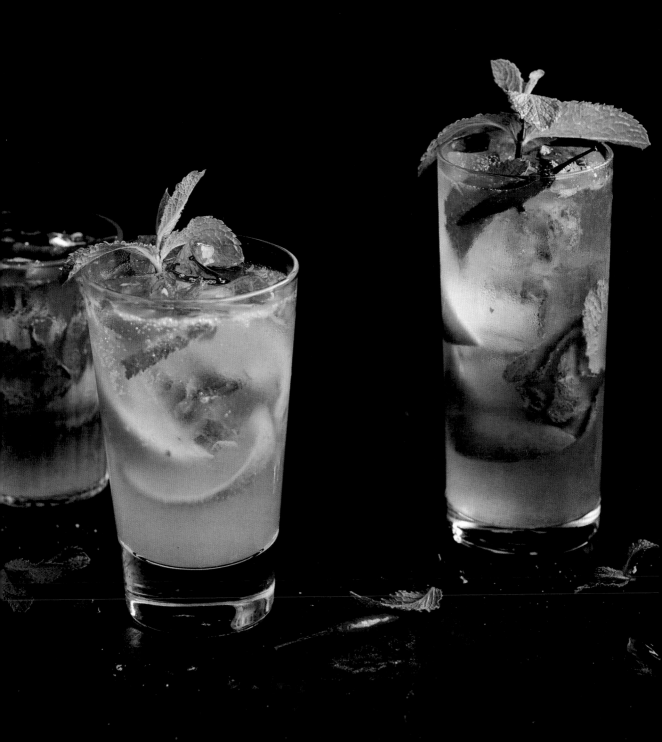

SPICY MOJITO

MAKES 4 GLASSES

4 highball glasses | Muddler or rolling pin

4 limes

24 fresh mint leaves, plus 4 sprigs
to serve

8 tsp superfine sugar

2 tsp Tabasco sauce

4 handfuls ice

2 cups white rum

2 cups soda water

4 fresh bird's eye chilies

Cut the limes into wedges and divide them between the glasses | Muddle (squash) them into the bottom of the glass to release the juices (be careful not to break the glass if it's thin)

Divide the mint leaves and the sugar among the glasses | Add the Tabasco sauce (use a little or a lot; this really depends on your palate) | Lightly crush everything together with the muddler to make sure the flavors are well mixed

Fill the glasses with ice | Pour the rum among them and stir everything together until the sugar has dissolved | Pick the leaves from the sprigs of mint

Put a little soda water into the glasses as a topper, garnish with fresh mint leaves, add a chili to each glass, and serve

GINGER & LEMONGRASS MOJITO

MAKES 4 GLASSES

Small saucepan | 4 highball glasses | Muddler or rolling pin

3 limes

24 fresh mint leaves, plus 4 sprigs
to serve

4 handfuls ice

2 cups white rum

2 cups club soda

4 sprigs fresh mint

FOR THE FLAVORED SYRUP

2-inch piece fresh ginger

3-inch lemongrass stalk

1 lime

6 tbsp sugar

6 tbsp water

First make the flavored syrup | Peel the ginger by scraping off the skin with a spoon and grate it into the saucepan | Trim the root of the lemongrass, peel away the tough outer layers, and chop into small pieces, then add to the pan | Cut the lime in half and squeeze in the juice, catching any seeds in your other hand | Add the sugar and water and stir everything together

Set the pan over medium heat for about 5 minutes, stirring all the time so the sugar dissolves | Take off the heat and set aside to cool to room temperature | Strain into a pitcher through a sieve

Cut the 3 limes into wedges and divide them among the glasses along with the mint leaves | Squash into the bottom of the glass with a muddler or the end of a rolling pin to release the juices (be careful not to break the glass if it's thin)

Put a handful of ice into each glass and pour a measure of rum and a measure of syrup into each one | Stir everything together | Add a splash of club soda into each glass and garnish with sprigs of fresh mint

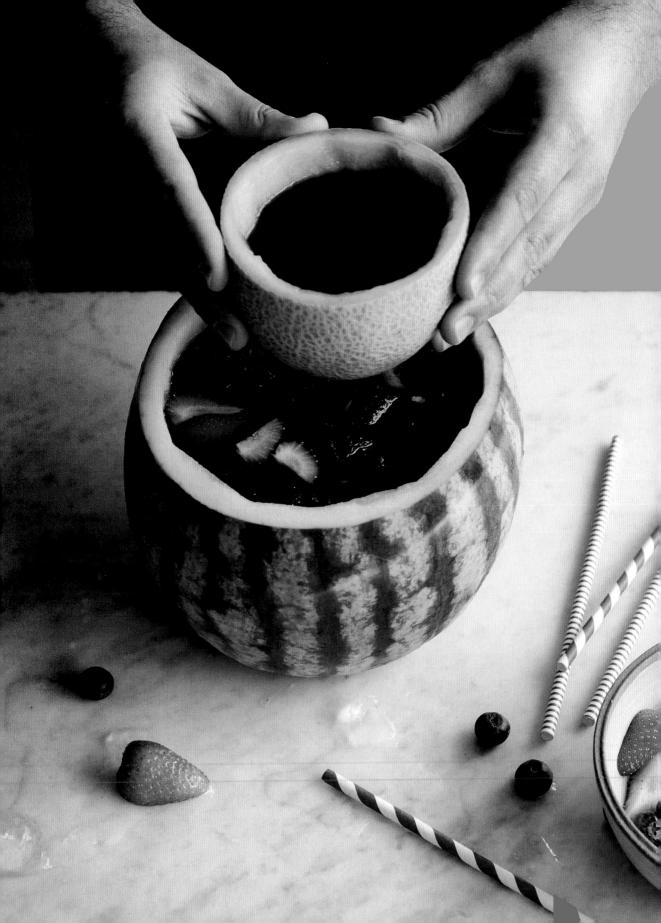

WATERMELON JÄGERBOMB PUNCH

We came up with this at the end of the first-ever BOSH! shoot. We had a watermelon, a Galia melon, energy drink, and a bottle of Jägermeister. We put the video live and it had 20 million views within a week! Use a really big watermelon and give the outside of the Galia melon a really good scrub before you put it inside.

SERVES 8

1 very large watermelon (at least 1½-ft diameter)
1 Galia melon (that will comfortably fit inside your watermelon)
2 cans (8 fl oz each) energy drink
8–12 ice cubes
handful fresh strawberries or blueberries
1½ cups Jägermeister

Stand blender or stick blender

Choose which side will be the bottom of the watermelon; if it doesn't stand up straight, use a knife to slice a very small sliver off the bottom | Once it's standing upright, cut horizontally across the middle | Take off the top and keep it for another recipe

Scoop out all the watermelon flesh and seeds from the bottom half until the inside looks neat | Transfer the flesh to the blender and blend (or use a stick blender and a bowl), then pour into a large bowl through a sieve to remove any seeds

Scrub the Galia melon with a brush to make sure it's clean | Lay it on its side and slice off the top 1½ inches| Scoop out the seeds and discard | Scoop out the melon flesh and transfer it to the blender | Whizz and then pour through a sieve into the bowl with the watermelon juice | Save the melon shell; this will act as your shot glass

Pour the energy drinks into the melon juice and stir | Now pour half the juice mixture into the hollowed-out watermelon | Carefully place the hollowed-out Galia melon into the middle of the watermelon so that it's floating in the melon juice

Drop ice cubes and berries into the melon juice around the edges | Pour the Jägermeister into the Galia melon (don't fill it too much in case it sinks) | Top up the edges with more melon juice to fill the watermelon bowl (you might have some left over, which you can use to refill later on)

Take the watermelon to the party, lift out the Galia "shot glass," and drop it back into the watermelon punch bowl in front of all your guests so that the Jägermeister spills into the melon juice | Wait for the applause

07

DESSERTS

Please your mouth with these
Scrumptious desserts and baked goods
To make your friends smile

SHIRLEY'S SHEFFIELD SCONES

Ian's mum, Shirley, always makes him a batch of these wonderful scones when he's back home. They are really tasty, easy, and incredibly addictive. The cashew clotted cream is amazing, and combined with the crumbly scones and sweet jam gives a flavor and texture sensation. Be careful not to overbake them; you're looking for a very light color.

MAKES 8

2 cups self-rising flour
3 tbsp + 1 tsp superfine sugar
½ tsp salt
2½ tbsp dairy-free butter or spread
½ cup unsweetened plant-based milk
⅓ cup golden raisins
raspberry jam, to serve

FOR THE CASHEW CREAM
5 oz cashews
1½ tbsp powdered sugar

Preheat oven to 390°F | Line a baking sheet | Small saucepan of boiling water | Food processor | Blender or hand mixer | Cooling rack

To make the cashew cream, put the cashews into the boiling water and cook for 15 minutes | Take off the heat, strain, and run under cold water to cool slightly | Put them into the blender with the powdered sugar and a splash of water and whizz to a thick cream (or use a hand mixer), adding more water if the mixture is too thick

Meanwhile, put the flour, superfine sugar, salt, dairy-free butter, and plant-based milk into the food processor and whizz to a dough | Take the blade out, tip in the raisins, and fold them into the mixture

Pull out roughly golf-ball-sized pieces of dough (about 1¼ inches each) and roll them into balls between your palms | Place on the lined baking sheet and squash until they're roughly ⅓ inch thick, leaving a little space between them as they will expand in the oven | Put the baking sheet in the oven and bake for roughly 12 minutes, until lightly golden | Remove and transfer to the cooling rack to cool

Serve the scones with a thin spread of dairy-free butter, a good dollop of raspberry jam, and the cashew clotted cream

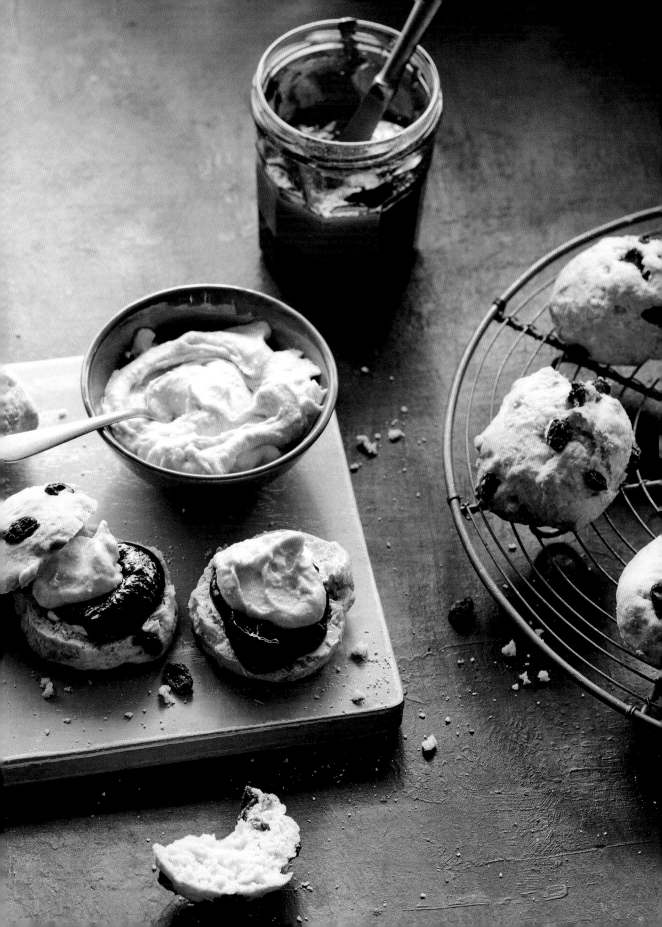

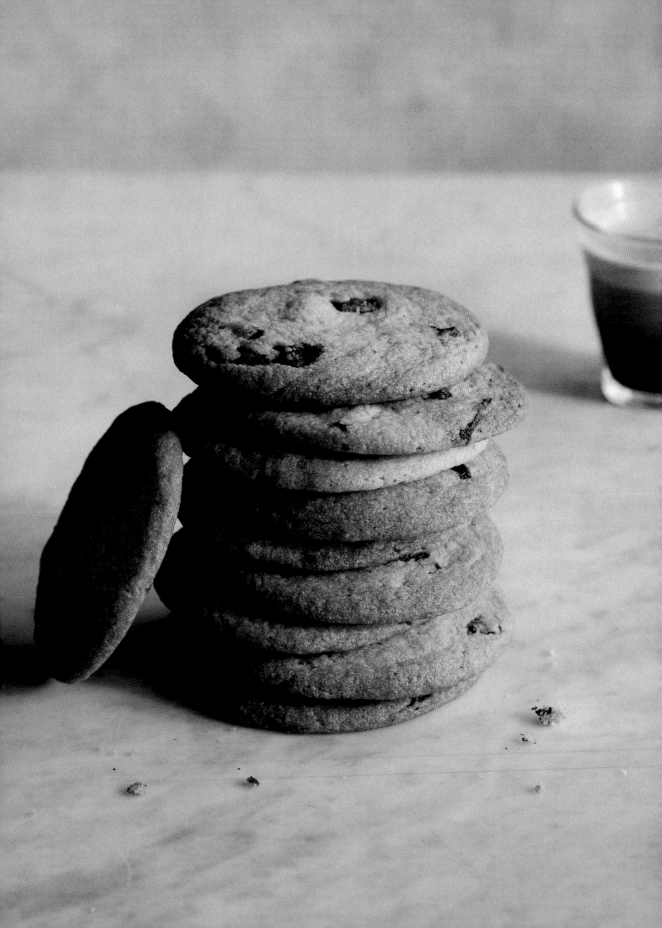

CHOCOLATE CHIP COOKIES

These are the perfect cookies—crunchy on the outside and gooey on the inside. Plus, they're incredibly easy to make and even easier if you use a food processor. Best served warm (of course), you could also add nuts, raisins, or dried fruit but, as self-confessed minimalists, we are perfectly happy with just the melted chocolate chips.

MAKES 25

1 cup + 1½ tbsp dairy-free butter or spread
1 cup + 3 tbsp superfine sugar
2 tsp vanilla extract
1 tbsp golden syrup
2⅓ cups all-purpose flour
1 tsp baking powder
½ tsp salt
3 oz dark chocolate

Preheat oven to 350°F | Line 2 baking sheets with parchment paper | Food processor, optional | Wire rack

Put the dairy-free butter, sugar, vanilla extract, and golden syrup into the food processor and whizz to a cream | Pour in the flour, baking powder, and salt and whizz everything together (you could also do all this in a big bowl with a wooden spoon) | Turn off the food processor and remove the blade | Chop the dark chocolate into small chips and fold them into the mixture with a spatula until they're evenly spread

Spoon walnut-sized pieces of the mixture onto the lined baking sheets, leaving 2 inches between them (you may need to cook them in batches) | Squash the balls to flatten them slightly (but not flat like pancakes)

Put the baking sheets in the oven and bake for 12–14 minutes, swapping racks halfway through so that they cook evenly | When they are ready the cookies should be golden around the edge, but paler in the middle | Take the baking sheets out of the oven but leave the cookies on them for 5–10 minutes to firm up a little, then transfer carefully to wire racks to cool

SPANISH BEACH CHURROS

We remember eating churros on the beach in Spain as kids and decided we needed to recreate the memory (even if we are in East London in the rain!). This is such an easy dish to make, you could even make a giant churros snake if you were feeling adventurous. Trust us, try this, you will thank us!

MAKES 12—15

1 cup sugar

2 tsp ground cinnamon

1½ quarts + 2 tbsp vegetable oil (preferably flavorless, like sunflower)

2 cups water

½ tsp salt

½ tsp vanilla extract

1¾ cups + 1 tbsp all-purpose flour

FOR THE CHOCOLATE SAUCE

3½ oz dark chocolate

¾ cup unsweetened plant-based milk

3 tbsp sugar

½ tsp vanilla extract

Small saucepan over low heat | 3 disposable piping bags or 1 clean reusable piping bag | ½-inch star tip | Large deep saucepan | Cooking thermometer, optional | Baking sheet lined with parchment paper | Medium saucepan | Line a large plate with a double layer of paper towels

First, make the chocolate sauce | Break up the chocolate and put it into the small saucepan with the plant-based milk, sugar, and vanilla | Stir to a smooth sauce | Transfer to a serving bowl | Set aside

Sprinkle ½ cup sugar and the cinnamon over a large plate and set aside

If you are using disposable piping bags, pile them up and roll them together to make one thick cone (a single bag is likely to split) | Cut a small hole at the tip, insert the piping tip, and push it all the way down to the bottom so that it sticks out of the hole | Spray or brush the inside of the bag with a little oil | If you are using a reusable bag, insert the tip and coat lightly with oil

Pour the 1½ quarts of oil into the large saucepan so that it comes a third of the way up the sides of the pan | Heat the oil to about 355°F, or until a wooden spoon dipped into the oil sizzles around the edges

Meanwhile, put the water, the remaining ½ cup sugar, the 2 tablespoons vegetable oil, salt, and vanilla extract into the medium saucepan and set over high heat | Bring to a boil, stirring to dissolve the sugar | Remove from the heat, add the flour, and beat vigorously with a wooden spoon until it forms a thick, sticky dough (you'll need to use a little elbow grease) | Spoon the mixture into the piping bag

Pipe 6 churros onto the lined baking sheet, each one about 4–6 inches long | Carefully transfer the churros to the hot oil (if you're feeling brave you can pipe them straight into the oil) | Fry for 8–10 minutes, until golden and cooked through | Use a wooden spoon to move them around if they stick together

Remove the churros with a slotted spoon and lay on the paper towels for 1 minute to drain | While they're still hot, transfer to the cinnamon sugar and roll until completely covered | Repeat with the remaining dough—you may need 3 or 4 batches | Serve with chocolate sauce

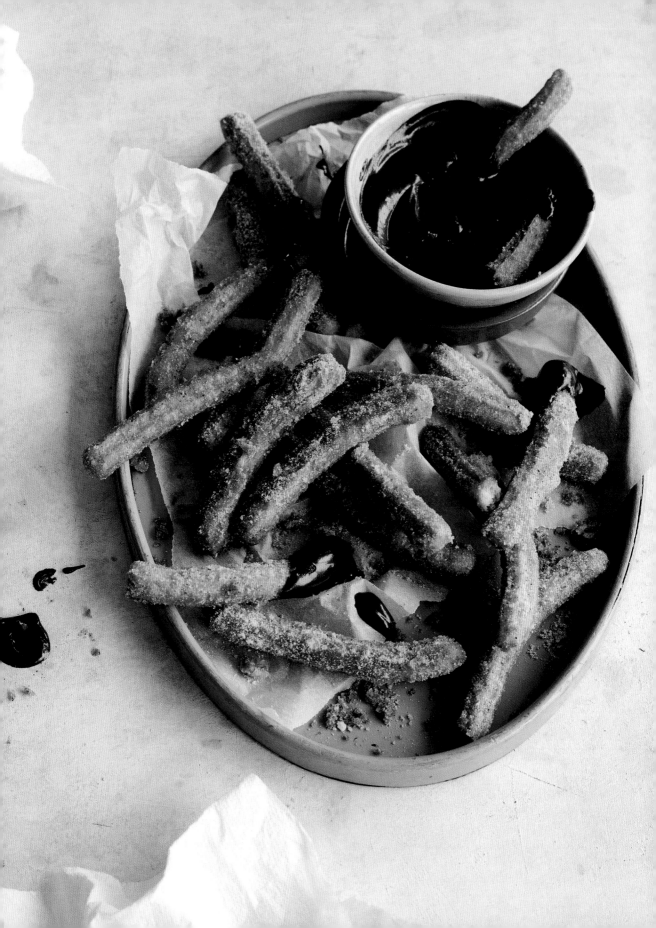

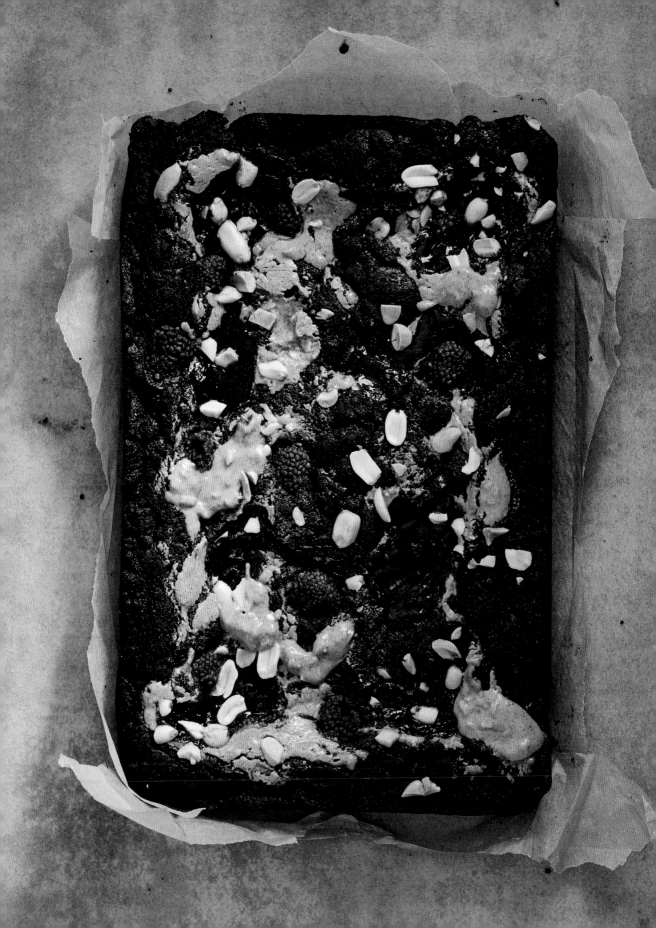

GOOEY PBJ BROWNIES

A surprising combination of two American classics—brownies and peanut butter and jelly. The tart, sweet jam contrasts with the earthy peanut and complements the sticky chocolate. Be careful not to overcook the outside—under is better than overdone with this one. For extra power-up points, serve with vegan ice cream and top with melted dark chocolate and nuts.

SERVES 12

2⅓ cups all-purpose flour

2¼ cups light muscovado sugar

⅔ cup cocoa powder

1 tsp baking powder

½ tsp salt

7½ tbsp smooth peanut butter
(thinner is better for this)

¾ cup + 3 tbsp water

¾ cup + 3 tbsp vegetable oil

2½ tbsp vanilla extract

1¾ oz dark chocolate

6 tbsp raspberry jam

3 oz raspberries

2 tbsp broken peanuts

Preheat oven to 320°F | 8 x 12-inch baking pan | Parchment paper | Food processor or electric mixer

Line the baking pan with the parchment paper, making sure there's a good overhang (this excess will act as handles to remove the brownie from the pan when it comes out of the oven)

Add the flour, sugar, cocoa, baking powder, and salt to the food processor and whizz to combine | Add 2 tbsp of the peanut butter, the water, oil, and vanilla | Blend until everything is well mixed (or put everything in a large mixing bowl and use an electric mixer) | Break the dark chocolate into squares and add it to the mixture | Blend for another few seconds to mix in the chocolate

Use a spatula or metal spoon to empty the brownie mix into the baking pan and smooth it out so it goes all the way to the edges of the pan | Use a spoon to pour and drag swirls of the remaining peanut butter and the jam randomly over the top of the brownie, decorating the whole top with long swirls of jam | Push the raspberries and peanuts randomly into the mixture

Put the pan in the hot oven and bake for 45 minutes, until cooked but still squidgy in the middle (try to avoid the outsides drying out and getting too browned; you want to take it out sooner than you think—the middle will still be soft and maybe even wobbly, but it will cool down to a gooey perfection)

Take the pan out of the oven and let it cool down almost to room temperature | Use the parchment paper to lift the brownie out of the pan and put it on a cutting board (you may need a friend to help with this to ensure it doesn't break in the middle) | Cut into brownie portions and serve

CARROT CAKE

Carrot cake is a favorite for many, and moist (what a word!) describes this version perfectly. It's sweet, wholesome, and as succulent a cake as you'll ever have tasted, with the perfect spice combination of cinnamon, nutmeg, and ginger and sweet, creamy icing. Decorate with walnuts to add the final bit of sizzle.

SERVES 8

4 medium carrots (about ¾ lb)
2 tbsp flaxseeds
6 tbsp warm water
2 cups minus 1 tbsp all-purpose flour
1 cup + 9 tbsp brown sugar
1½ tsp baking powder
1½ tsp baking soda
2 tsp ground cinnamon
2 tsp ground nutmeg
1 tsp ground ginger
2 tsp vanilla extract
½ cup vegetable oil
1 tbsp apple cider vinegar
¼ tsp salt
½ cup unsweetened plant-based milk
½ cup golden raisins
1¾ oz walnut halves
zest of 1 lemon

FOR THE ICING
5½ tbsp dairy-free butter or spread at
    room temperature, plus extra for
    greasing
1 tbsp vanilla extract
3¾ cups powdered sugar
½ lemon

Preheat oven to 350°F | 7-inch deep cake pan with a removable bottom | Parchment paper | Food processor or electric mixer

Lay the bottom of the cake pan on the parchment paper and draw a circle around it; cut it out | Grease the inside of the pan with dairy-free butter, lay the paper round in the bottom, and then grease some more

Trim and finely grate the carrots | Put the flaxseeds into a small bowl, add the warm water, and stir them around until you have a smooth paste | Leave for 5 minutes to thicken

Put the flour, sugar, baking powder, baking soda, cinnamon, nutmeg, and ginger into the food processor | Add the vanilla extract, vegetable oil, apple cider vinegar, salt, and plant-based milk, along with the flaxseed paste | Whizz to a batter (or beat everything together in a large mixing bowl with an electric mixer for 2–3 minutes)

Pour the batter into a mixing bowl | Add the raisins and the grated carrot and fold everything together | Pour the batter into the pan and put the pan in the oven | Bake for 50–55 minutes, until a skewer inserted into the center of the cake comes out clean | Take the cake out of the oven and let it cool to room temperature

Meanwhile, clean the food processor or electric mixer | Now make the icing | Put the dairy-free butter, vanilla extract, and powdered sugar into the food processor or a clean bowl | Squeeze the lemon juice into the bowl, catching any seeds in your other hand | Whizz to a cream that is thick but spreadable

Cut the cake in half horizontally and spread a third of the frosting over the bottom layer | Sandwich with the top half and spread the rest of the frosting over the top of the cake | Decorate with the walnut halves and lemon zest | The cake will keep in the fridge for up to 3 days

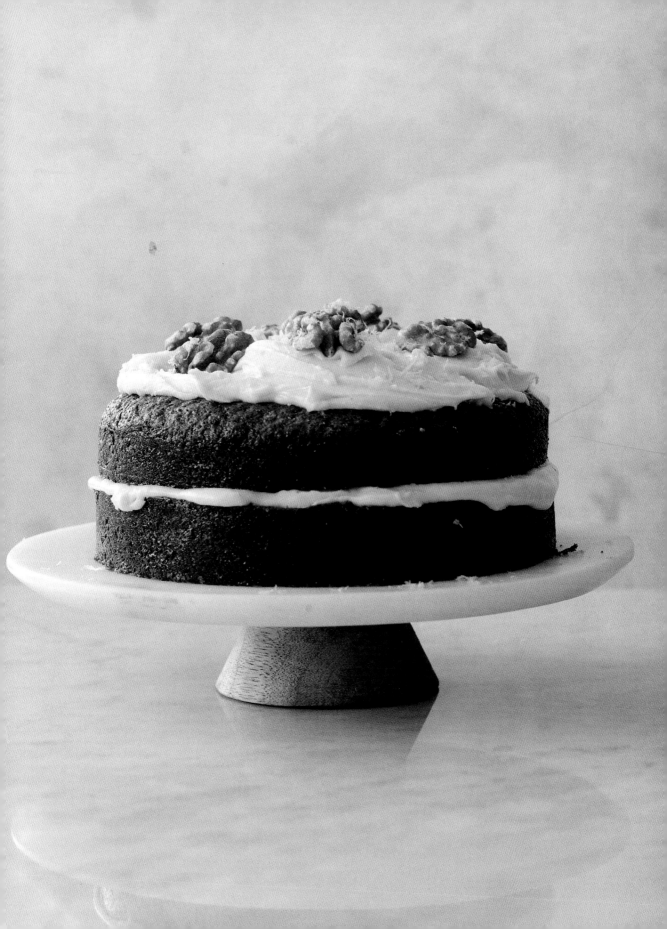

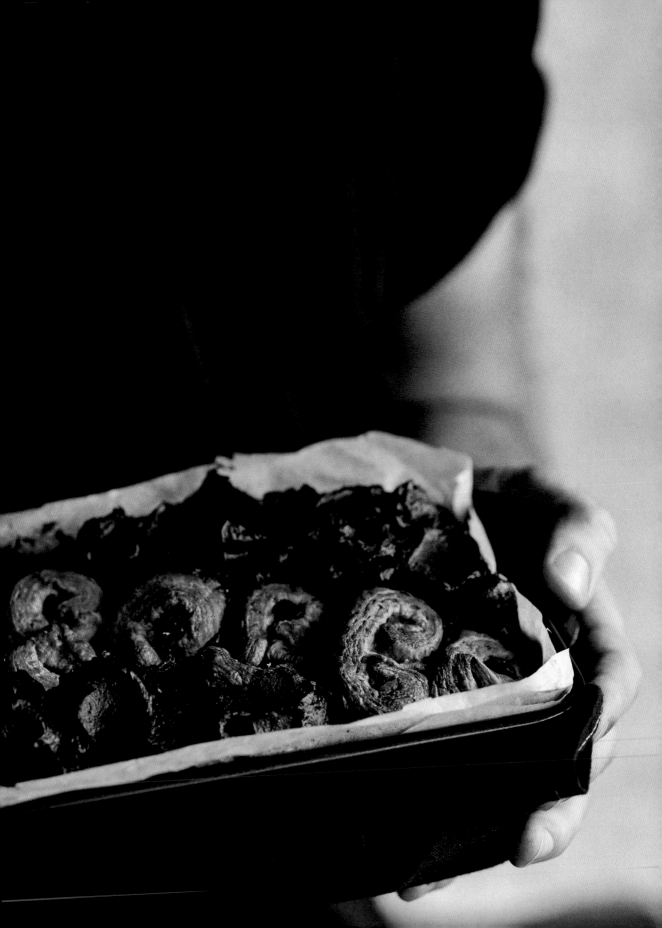

PAIN AU CHOCOLAT LOAF CAKE

This is the most ridiculous thing we could think to do with ready-to-bake dairy-free chocolate croissants. It's silly, zany, fun, and tasty, and watching the croissants rise in the oven makes you feel like a kid again. Be sure to skewer them so they stay nice and straight while they bake.

SERVES 8

FOR THE CAKE
6 ready-to-bake vegan chocolate croissants
1½ cups all-purpose flour
1 cup superfine sugar
3 tbsp cocoa powder
2 tsp baking soda
½ tsp salt
5 tbsp vegetable oil
1½ tsp vanilla extract
1½ tsp distilled white vinegar
½ cup water
½ cup unsweetened plant-based milk

FOR THE ICING
¾ cup powdered sugar
5 tbsp cocoa powder
2 tbsp dairy-free butter or spread, plus a little extra for greasing
1 tbsp + 2 tsp unsweetened plant-based milk
½ tsp vanilla extract

Preheat oven to 320°F | 2-lb loaf pan | Parchment paper | Long wooden skewer | Food processor or electric hand mixer

Line the loaf pan by cutting a strip of parchment paper that is a little longer and wider than the bottom of the pan, so you can use the parchment to pull out the cake when it's ready | Grease the inside of the pan with a little dairy-free butter

Prepare the chocolate croissants following the instructions on the package | Line them up down the middle of the loaf pan, standing them on their ends | Rest the skewer on top of the pan, following the line of pastries and resting the tips on either end | Carefully twist the skewer into and through the top of the first pain au chocolat to attach it | Repeat with all the pastries until they're attached to the skewer | The skewer gives the pastries stability and keeps them standing upright

Put all the rest of the ingredients for the cake into the food processor and whizz to a batter (or put into a mixing bowl and beat together for 2–3 minutes with an electric hand mixer)

Pour the cake mixture evenly down each side of the pan (it should fill the pan to about three-quarters full) | Cover the pan with foil and put it in the hot oven | Bake for 30 minutes, then remove the foil, put it back in the oven, and bake for 20–25 minutes longer, until the cake is firm and a skewer inserted into the middle comes out clean (this additional cooking will give the pains au chocolat a lovely crispy top) | Remove from the oven and leave to cool in the pan | Clean out the food processor

Once the cake has cooled to room temperature, lift it out of the pan with the parchment paper and lay it on a serving plate | Remove the skewer

Put all the icing ingredients into the clean food processor and whizz to a thick, rich icing | Carefully spread the icing over the cake part of the loaf (don't spread it on the pains au chocolat) | Leave to firm up and serve

ULTIMATE CHOCOLATE FUDGE CAKE

Inspired by our most popular video ever, this is arguably the greatest chocolate cake we've ever tasted. Easy to make and delicious to eat, it's perfect birthday-cake fodder. Just make sure you have a gym membership, as this one is super indulgent. How naughty? Very naughty. Go on. Do it.

SERVES 8

¾ cup + 3 tbsp all-purpose flour
½ cup + 2 tbsp cocoa powder
1½ tbsp baking powder
1 tsp vanilla extract
1 cup maple syrup
1½ cups unsweetened plant-based milk
dairy-free butter or spread, for greasing

FOR THE CHOCOLATE ICING
½ cup + 2 tbsp cocoa powder
2⅔ cups powdered sugar
4 tbsp dairy-free butter or spread
1 tsp vanilla extract
¼ cup + 1 tsp unsweetened plant-based
  milk

Preheat oven to 350°F | Two 8-inch cake pans | Parchment paper | Food processor or electric mixer | Cooling rack | Spatula or long smooth knife

Lay the cake pans on the parchment paper and draw circles around the bottoms, then cut out the rounds | Grease the inside of the pans with dairy-free butter and lay the paper rounds in the bottom | Grease with more dairy-free butter

First make the cake | Put the flour, cocoa powder, baking powder, vanilla extract, maple syrup, and plant-based milk into the food processor and whizz to a batter (or put in a bowl and whisk with the electric mixer for 1–2 minutes)

Pour half the cake batter into each pan, making sure it is divided equally | Put the pans in the oven on the middle rack and bake for 25 minutes | Don't worry if the tops of the cakes crack a little while baking; this will all be covered in icing later | Wash the food processor

Take the cakes out of the oven and let them cool to room temperature in the pans | The layers will be quite fragile, so carefully turn them out of the pans onto the cooling rack and put the rack in the refrigerator for at least 30 minutes (this will make the icing process easier)

To make the icing, put the cocoa powder, powdered sugar, dairy-free butter, vanilla extract, and plant-based milk into the food processor and whizz to a really thick, smooth icing (or put them in a bowl and whisk with the electric mixer)

Take one layer of the cake and put it on a large plate | Cover the top with a third of the chocolate icing | Lay the second cake on top | Cover the whole cake with the rest of the icing | Put the cake in the fridge for 1 hour to firm up | Remove the cake from the fridge, cut it into slices, and serve

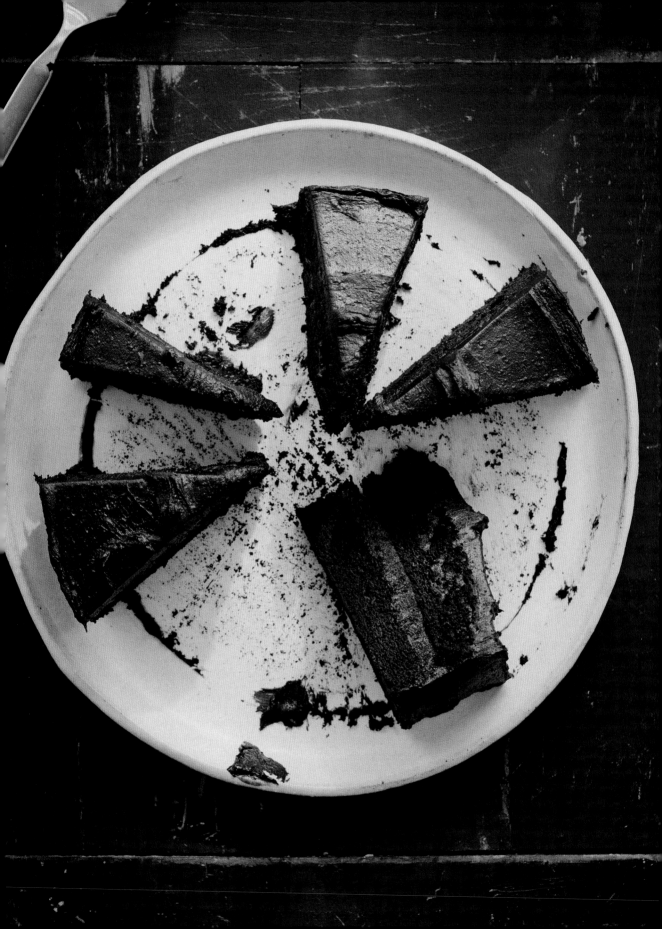

AQUAFABA CHOCOLATE MOUSSE

This is effortlessly simple and yet one of the most delicious chocolate mousses we've ever tasted. Decadent and luxurious, it's made with a handful of ingredients and can be prepared in advance and left in the fridge for later. The magical thrill of the aquafaba transformation (and the ensuing conversations with your guests!) is really something.

SERVES 3

Medium saucepan over high heat | Heatproof bowl | Electric mixer

3½ oz dark chocolate
liquid from 1 can (15 oz) chickpeas
    (aquafaba, 1 generous ½ cup)
2½ tbsp sugar
1 tsp vanilla extract
pinch of salt
handful blueberries, to serve

Pour 1¼ inches water into the pan and bring to a boil | Reduce the heat to a simmer | Put a heatproof bowl on top of the pan, ensuring the water doesn't touch the bottom | Break 3 oz of the dark chocolate into the bowl and leave it to melt | Remove and leave to cool a little

Pour the aquafaba into a large bowl and use the electric mixer (a hand whisk won't cut it this time) to whisk the liquid for 10–15 minutes—it will gradually firm up, as if by magic | Stop when the mixture makes stiff peaks if you lift out the beaters | Gently fold in the melted chocolate, sugar, vanilla, and salt using a large metal spoon or spatula, making sure you don't beat out too much air

Spoon the mousse into serving glasses or bowls and chill for 2 hours

Grate the remaining ½ oz chocolate | Dress the individual mousses with a handful of blueberries and a touch of grated chocolate just before serving

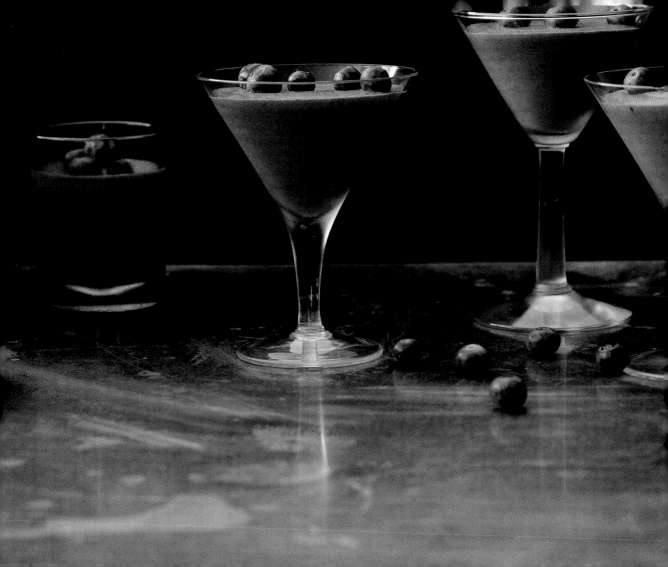

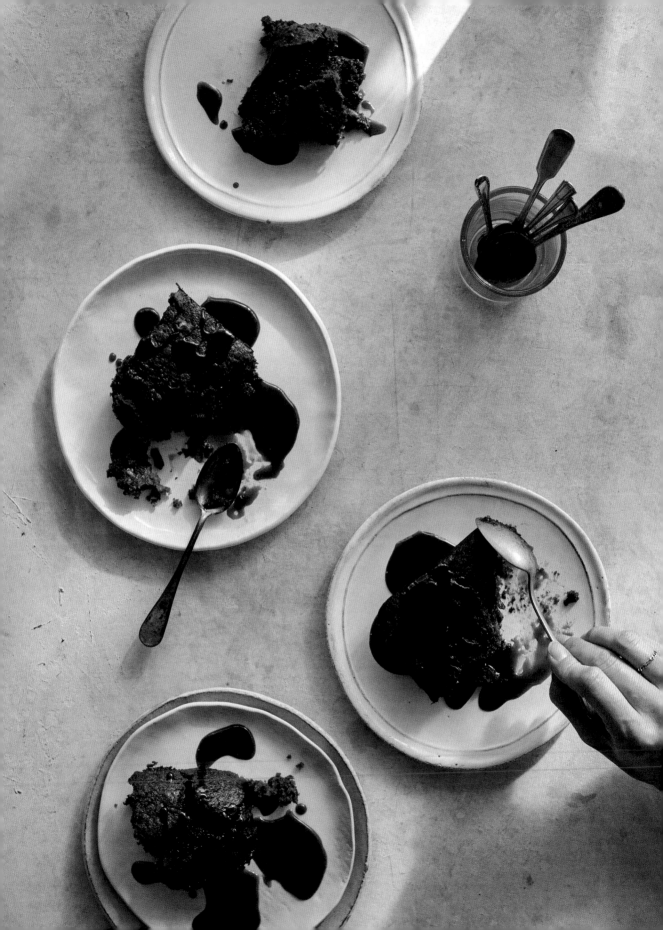

STICKY TOFFEE PUDDING

It's hard to describe just how good this dish is. You have to try it. It's just like Grandma used to make: incredibly smoky and toffee-and-caramel-flavored. The notes of cinnamon, ginger, and nutmeg add hints of deliciousness to the orgy of richness. This dish goes really well with a serving of dairy-free ice cream!

SERVES 6

6 oz dates
1½ cups unsweetened plant-based milk
1 tsp vanilla extract
1½ tsp baking soda
8 tbsp + 7 tbsp dairy-free butter or spread
1 cup dark brown sugar
generous ¾ cup self-rising flour
½ tsp ground nutmeg
1 tsp ground ginger
1 tsp ground cinnamon
1 tsp salt
1 tbsp golden syrup
3 tbsp coconut cream

Preheat oven to 320°F | Small saucepan over medium heat | 10 x 6 x 2-inch ovenproof dish greased with dairy-free butter

Cut the dates into small pieces, removing the pits as you go | Put them in the saucepan along with the plant-based milk and vanilla extract and cook until the dates are soft, about 10 minutes

Take the pan off the heat and stir in the baking soda | Let the liquid cool to room temperature | Add 8 tbsp of the dairy-free butter and ½ cup of the sugar | Add the flour, nutmeg, ginger, cinnamon, and salt, and stir them a few times with a spoon until just combined, but not overmixed

Pour the mixture into the greased baking dish, put the dish in the oven, and bake for 35–40 minutes, until risen and a skewer inserted into the center comes out clean

Meanwhile, clean the saucepan and put it back over medium heat | Put the golden syrup, the remaining ½ cup brown sugar, and the remaining 7 tbsp dairy-free butter into the pan, stir, and reduce the heat to low | Cook for 5 minutes until you have a syrup | Remove the pan from the burner, allow it to cool slightly, and then stir in the coconut cream | Pour into a small pitcher

To serve, use a knife to cut the sticky toffee pudding into slices | Place each slice into a bowl and cover with the delicious toffee drizzle | Serve and enjoy!

MIXED BERRY CRUMBLE

This crumble is luxuriously fruity, crumbly, and crunchy.
It's easy to make and great to share, perfect for a cool-
season dessert. You can, of course, use any berries that are
in season for this; we've opted for a mixed berry selection.
A little dairy-free oat cream or custard would work perfectly
with this dessert.

SERVES 6–8

2¼ lb mixed berries, such as
   blackberries, raspberries,
   strawberries, and blueberries
⅓ cup + ½ cup superfine sugar
1 tsp vanilla extract
3 tbsp cornstarch
1¾ cups whole wheat flour
generous 2¾ cups rolled oats
1 tsp ground cinnamon
1 cup (8 oz) dairy-free butter or spread
dairy-free custard or oat cream,
   to serve, optional

Preheat oven to 350°F | 12 x 8-inch baking dish

Put the berries, ⅓ cup of the sugar, the vanilla extract, and cornstarch into a large mixing bowl and mix together, making sure all the fruit is covered in the sugar and cornstarch | Tip into the baking dish and smooth the top with the back of a spoon

Place the flour, oats, and cinnamon in a bowl and mix well | Scoop small pieces of the dairy-free butter into the bowl with a spoon and then get your hands in and pinch and rub everything together with your fingertips until it looks like breadcrumbs | Add the remaining ½ cup sugar and mix well | Scatter the crumble mixture evenly all over the berry filling, covering it all the way to the edges

Put the dish in the hot oven and bake for 50 minutes, or until the top is golden and the fruit is bubbling up around the edges of the dish | Take out of the oven and serve with the dairy-free custard or oat cream, if you like

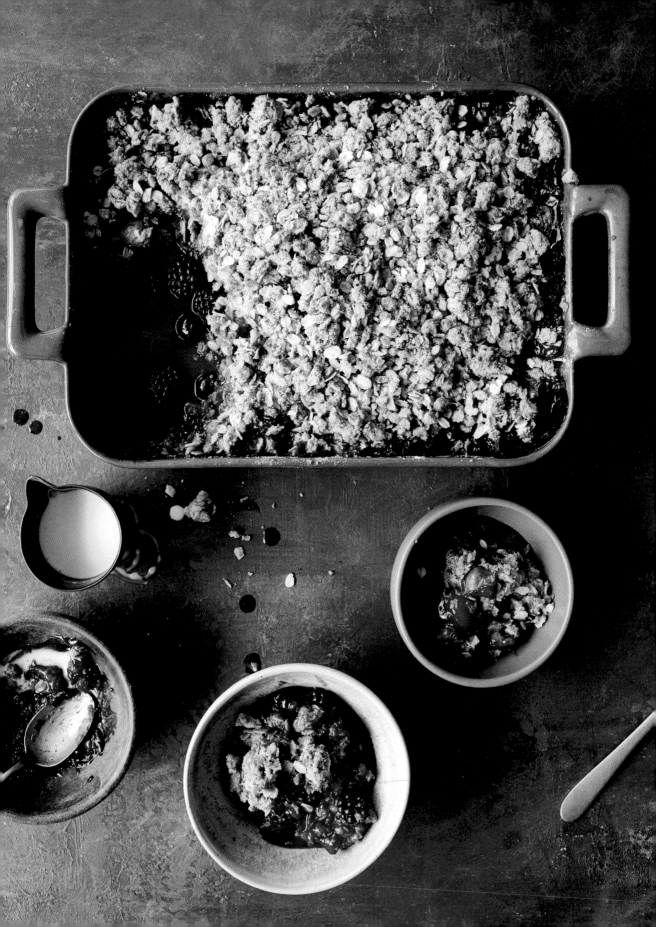

SALTED CARAMEL CHOCOLATE CRUNCH TART

Oozing with sugary, crunchy, caramel, chocolatey goodness, this insanely tasty dish has everything you could want from a dessert. It is regularly showcased at events since we're so proud of it, and it's got that "pick-up-and-go" factor, so would sit comfortably in a buffet. This is the dish you'll want to make again and again.

SERVES 10

1 package refrigerated dairy-free pie dough
¾ cup coconut cream
2⅔ cups light brown sugar
2 tsp sea salt
7 oz hazelnuts
3½ oz pecans
3½ oz dark chocolate
2 tsp vanilla extract

Preheat oven to 350°F | Line a pie tin or small rimmed baking sheet with parchment paper | Medium saucepan

Unroll the dough onto the lined pie tin or baking sheet, making sure the edges of the pastry fold up the sides of the sheet and pressing it into the corners | Chill in the freezer for 10 minutes to stop the pastry from shrinking and the sides from collapsing

Put the pastry in the hot oven and bake for about 30 minutes, or until golden brown (it will bubble a bit but don't worry, those bubbles will deflate) | Take the pan out of the oven

Meanwhile, set the saucepan over medium heat | Pour in the coconut cream and stir so that it becomes completely liquid | Pour in the sugar and stir continuously for at least 5 minutes, until the mixture thickens and darkens in color | Sprinkle in the salt and stir it into the caramel

Put the hazelnuts and pecans into a mortar and break them up with the pestle (or put them in a plastic bag and bash them with a rolling pin) | Tip the broken nuts into the pan and stir them in so that they're well covered in the sticky caramel sauce | Break the chocolate into the pan and stir until it has melted into the caramel and the nuts are completely covered | Take the pan off the heat, stir in the vanilla extract, and set aside

Pour the chocolate caramel into the pastry shell and spread it out to the edges | Smooth the top with an offset spatula or smooth knife | Put the tart back in the oven for 3 minutes, then take it out and let it cool to room temperature in the pan | Put the cooled tart in the fridge for 30 minutes to cool down and firm up

Take the tart out of the fridge and carefully remove it from the pan | Cut into slices and serve

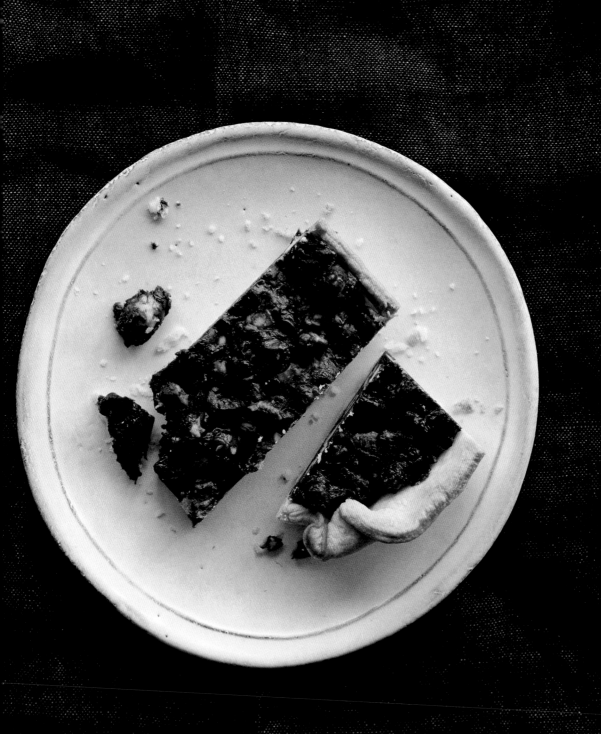

APPLE PEAR PIE

Who doesn't like a slice of warm apple pie? The cinnamon and apple flavors go together perfectly and complement the contrasting crispy crust and sweet, fruity center. This one's pretty easy to prepare, made much easier by using store-bought pie dough. Everyone should have a good apple pie in their repertoire. This can be yours!

SERVES 6

Two 9-inch refrigerated dairy-free
    pie crusts
1¾ lb apples
1 lb pears
½ lemon
3 tbsp superfine sugar
2 tbsp maple syrup
2 tsp ground cinnamon
2 tbsp all-purpose flour
small pinch of salt
2 tbsp unsweetened plant-based milk
1 tbsp brown sugar
soy cream, optional, to serve

Preheat oven to 350°F | Heavy baking sheet in oven | Board dusted with flour | Clear some space in the fridge | 9-inch deep-dish tart or pie tin | Pastry brush

Lay one of the pie crusts inside the pie tin | Press it neatly into the edges and all the way up the sides and just over the top edge, making sure there's no trapped air | Cut away the excess pastry and use pieces to patch up any gaps | Set the second pie crust aside on a floured board

Put the pie shell in the fridge for 15 minutes to chill along with the second pie crust on the board (this will stop it shrinking in the oven)

Meanwhile, peel and core the apples and pears and cut them roughly into ⅓-inch chunks | Put them in a large bowl and squeeze over the juice of the lemon, catching any seeds in your other hand | Add the superfine sugar, maple syrup, cinnamon, flour, and salt and mix together with a wooden spoon

Spread the apple mixture evenly into the chilled pie shell | Lay the top crust over the top and crimp the edges by pinching all around the rim between your thumb and forefinger, or by squashing the top and bottom crusts together with a fork | Cut off any excess pastry with a sharp knife

Put the pie tin on top of the hot baking sheet in the oven and bake for 40 minutes, then take it out of the oven | Brush the pie with the plant-based milk, sprinkle it with brown sugar, and put it back in the oven for 10–12 minutes, or until it's crisp and golden on top

Take the pie out of the oven | Let it cool down for at least 15 minutes before serving with soy cream, if using

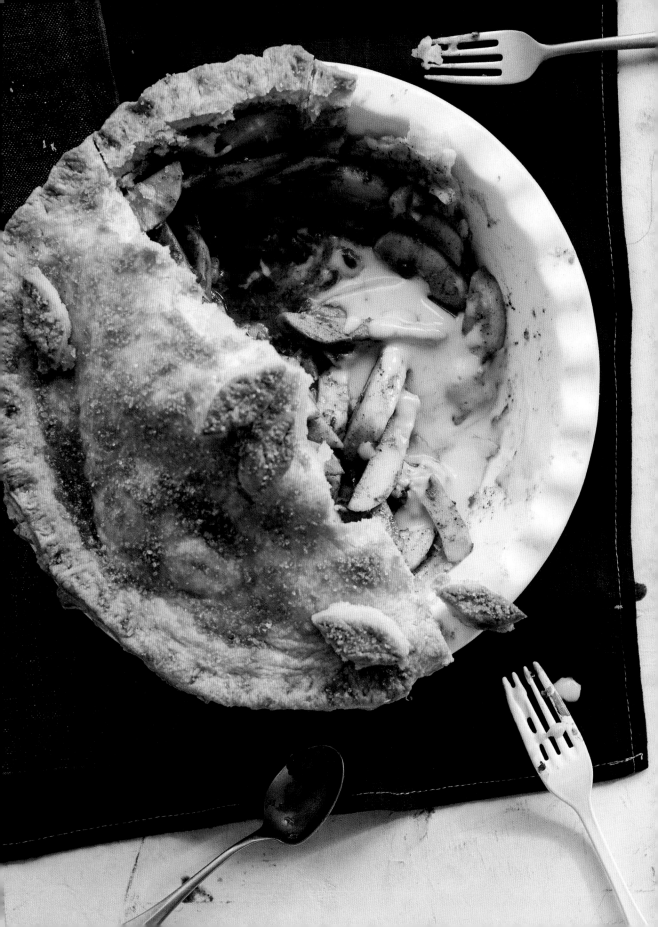

08

BREAKFASTS

From daily smoothies
To weekly bowls of goodness
Start your day right here

BANANA PANCAKES

We had to include some banana pancakes! This is a wonderful easy-to-prepare breakfast for those mornings when you are looking for something delicious and impressive to start your day. Experiment with toppings, but if you make sure there is plenty of fruit it counts as one of your five (or ten) a day!

SERVES 2

1½ ripe bananas
½ tbsp coconut oil, plus extra for frying
½ tsp ground cinnamon
⅔ cup all-purpose flour
1 tbsp superfine sugar
1 tsp baking powder
1 cup unsweetened plant-based milk
1 oz pecans
3 tbsp maple syrup
¾ oz dark chocolate

Preheat oven to warm | Ovenproof plate | Food processor | Frying pan over medium-high heat

Put one banana, the coconut oil, cinnamon, flour, sugar, baking powder, and plant-based milk into the food processor and whizz to a smooth batter | Add a little coconut oil to the frying pan and warm it so that it's reasonably hot, but not smoking

Pour about 3 tablespoons of the mixture for each pancake you can fit into the pan and fry for about 2 minutes, until bubbles start to appear on the surface of the pancakes | Flip them over and fry the other sides for another 1–2 minutes | Remove to the ovenproof plate and put it in the oven to keep warm while you cook the rest of the pancakes

Slice the ½ banana | Put the pecans in a mortar and lightly crush with a pestle (or put them in a plastic bag and crush with a rolling pin)

Stack the pancakes on 2 serving plates | Put the banana slices on top and sprinkle on the pecans | Drizzle with lashings of maple syrup and grate the chocolate over

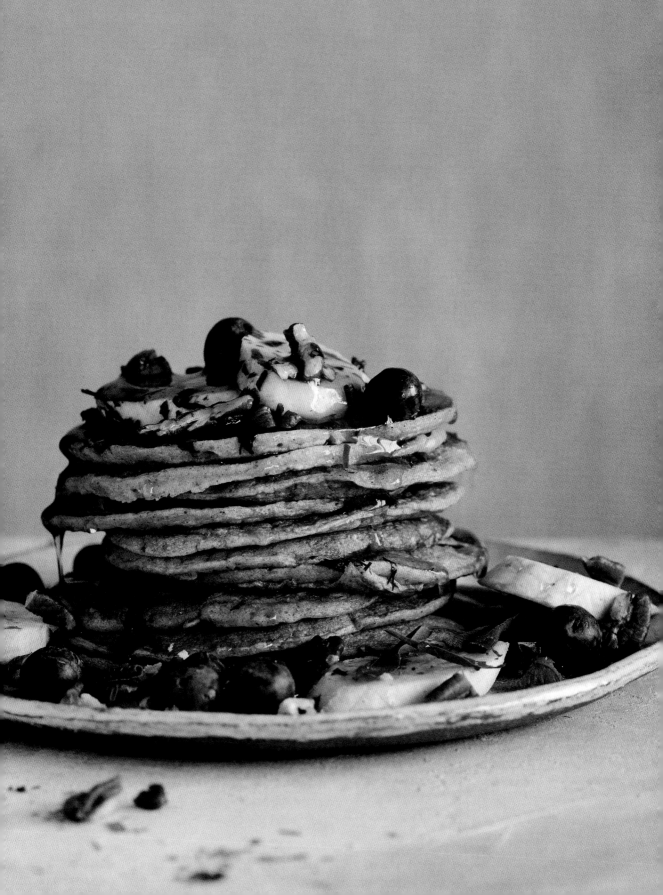

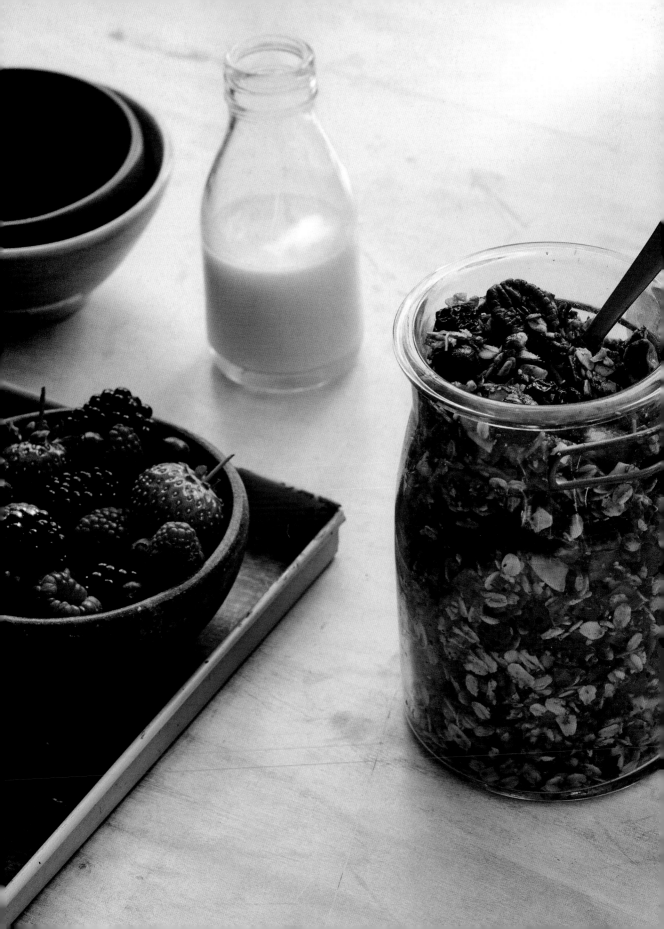

CHOCOLATE GRANOLA

Remember how chocolate cereal used to make the milk go chocolatey? Well this incredibly moreish dish has that in abundance. It makes a fantastic breakfast, but would also work as a replacement for popcorn on movie night. For a healthier (but still tasty) version, omit the sugar.

SERVES 6–8

2 oz Brazil nuts
2 oz pecans
2 oz hazelnuts
2½ oz coconut flakes
½ tsp sea salt
3¾ cups oats
¼ cup coconut sugar
½ cup + 3 tbsp coconut oil
5 tsp maple syrup
1 tsp vanilla extract
1¾ oz dark chocolate
6 tbsp raisins

Preheat oven to 280°F | Line a large baking sheet | Large saucepan over very low heat

Put all the nuts in the middle of a clean kitchen towel, wrap them up, and break them with a rolling pin so that they are about the size of raisins | Tip the broken nuts into a mixing bowl | Add the coconut flakes, salt, oats, and coconut sugar and mix everything together with a wooden spoon

Slowly melt the coconut oil in the saucepan | Add the maple syrup and vanilla extract and mix everything together | Pour the dry ingredients from the bowl into the saucepan and mix it all together

Pour the granola onto the lined baking sheet (the wider the pan, the crunchier the granola) | Put the pan in the oven and bake for 40 minutes

Take the pan out of the oven | Break the dark chocolate into small chunks the size of chocolate chips and sprinkle them over the granola along with the raisins | Leave to cool to room temperature

Break up the granola into bite-sized chunks and transfer to an airtight container | Enjoy your delicious granola with lashings of plant-based milk and chopped fresh fruit

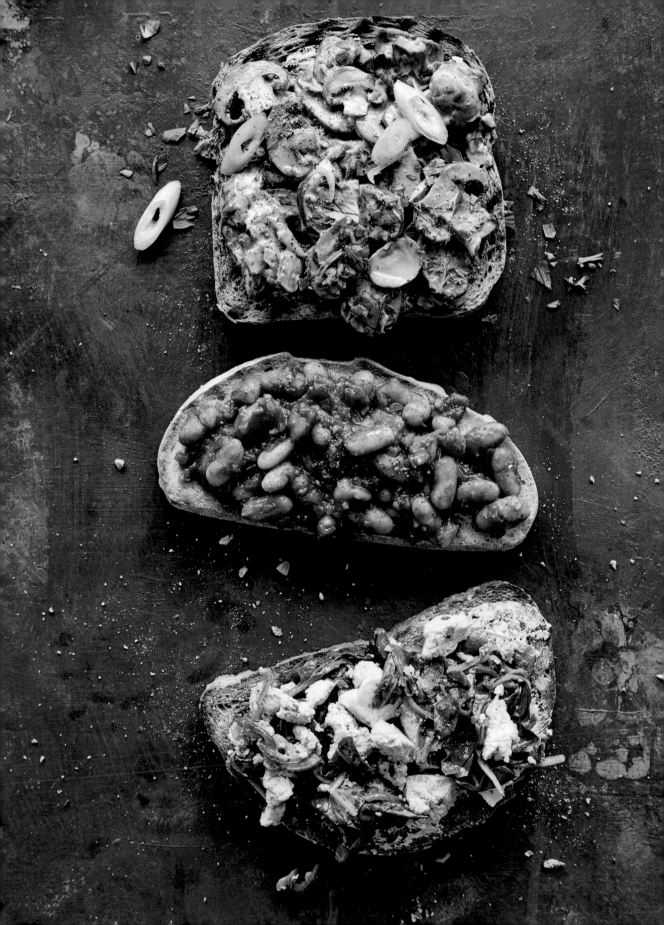

BOSH! BREAKFAST TOASTS

The humble slice of bread, toasted to perfection, is a mighty meal to behold. Here are three of our favorite ways to enjoy a quick-fix mini English breakfast. They're most delicious with quality sourdough bread that brings additional flavor to the meal, even better if it's from a real baker! The better the bread, the better the breakfast.

CREAMY GARLIC MUSHROOM TOAST

So. Rich. So. Creamy. Cannot. Compute. This garlicky mushroom dish is effortless and full of voluptuous, creamy flavors.

SERVES 2

12 oz mushrooms
2 small garlic cloves
2 scallions
1 tbsp olive oil
2 large or 4 small slices
    good-quality fresh bread
1½ tbsp dairy-free butter or spread,
    plus extra for spreading
5 tbsp soy cream
small handful fresh parsley leaves
salt and black pepper

Large frying pan over medium-high heat | Toaster or broiler

Slice the mushrooms | Peel and mince the garlic | Trim the roots and ends from the scallions and finely slice

Put the olive oil in the pan | Add the mushrooms and cook for 10 minutes | Add the garlic and three-quarters of the scallions (saving some of the green ends for garnish) | Cook for 3 minutes

Put the bread in the toaster or under the broiler

Add the dairy-free butter to the pan of mushrooms and stir it in until it melts | Pour the soy cream into the pan and stir it into the mushrooms | Take the pan off the heat | Season to taste with salt and pepper

Roughly chop the parsley and stir most of it into the mushrooms | Take the toast out of the toaster or broiler and spread it with dairy-free butter | Divide the mushroom mixture equally among the toasts | Sprinkle with the remaining scallions and parsley | Grind over a little black pepper and serve immediately

SMOKY BBQ BEANS ON TOAST

These homemade BBQ beans are a revelation. They're smoky, rich, and incredibly punchy, plus they're filled with protein. Feel free to adjust the chili to suit your taste.

SERVES 2

Medium saucepan over medium heat | Toaster or broiler

½ onion
2 garlic cloves
1 tbsp olive oil
1 tbsp tomato paste
¼ tsp smoked paprika
¼ tsp chili powder
¼ tsp dried thyme
1 tbsp light brown sugar
1 tbsp light soy sauce
1 can (15 oz) cannellini beans
2 large or 4 small slices
    good-quality fresh bread
7 tbsp tomato puree
dairy-free butter or spread, for spreading
fresh parsley leaves, to garnish,
    optional
salt and black pepper

Peel and finely chop the onion and garlic | Add the olive oil to the pan | Add the onion and garlic and stir until the onion is translucent and soft, about 10 minutes

Add the tomato paste, smoked paprika, chili powder, thyme, sugar, and soy sauce and stir them into the onions | Cook for 2 minutes

Drain and rinse the cannellini beans, then add them to the pan | Stir them around so that they're covered in the sauce | Cook for another 2–3 minutes

Put the bread in the toaster or under the broiler

Pour the tomato puree into the pan and let it simmer until the sauce has thickened, about 5 minutes | Chop the parsley, if using

Taste the sauce and season it with pepper and a little salt | Take the toast out of the toaster or broiler and spread it with dairy-free butter | Put the beans on top, sprinkle with the parsley, if using, and serve immediately

TOFU SCRAMBLE ON TOAST

This version of the classic scramble uses tofu as a base and is spongy, crumbly, and super satisfying. Added to our Big Breakfast (see page 265), it would create a meal for a king and queen.

(see page 265)

SERVES 2

½ small red onion
1 garlic clove
2 oz baby spinach
2 tbsp olive oil
1 block (10 oz) extra-firm tofu
2 tsp dairy-free butter or spread,
    plus more for spreading
1 tbsp nutritional yeast
1 tsp ground turmeric
½ tsp chili flakes
2 large or 4 small slices
    good-quality fresh bread
salt and black pepper

Large frying pan over medium heat | Toaster or broiler

Peel and finely slice the onion and garlic | Roughly chop the spinach

Add the olive oil to the pan | Add the onions and garlic and cook until the onions are well softened, about 10 minutes | Crumble the tofu into the pan along with the 2 teaspoons of dairy-free butter | Add the nutritional yeast, turmeric, and chili flakes and stir everything together | Cook for around 5 minutes | Season with salt and pepper

Put the bread in the toaster or under the broiler

Add the spinach to the pan and stir until well wilted, another 1–2 minutes | Taste again and season if necessary

Take the toast out of the toaster or broiler and spread it with dairy-free butter | Top it with the spinach and scramble, grind over some black pepper and serve immediately

BANANA BREAD

Is it a dessert? Is it a breakfast? We can't decide. Is it tasty? Hell yes. Want to know what makes this amazing recipe even better? Spread some peanut butter on top. Oh my goodness it's insane. Or dairy-free ice cream to turn it into a whopper of a dessert.

MAKES 1 LOAF

scant 2 cups all-purpose flour
6 tbsp light brown sugar
6 tbsp granulated sugar
1½ tbsp cocoa powder
½ tsp baking soda
½ tsp salt
½ tsp ground allspice
7 tbsp + 2 tsp dairy-free butter or spread
3 ripe bananas
¼ cup almond milk
2 tbsp maple syrup
1 tsp apple cider vinegar
1 tsp vanilla extract
2 oz dark chocolate
1¾ oz pecans

Preheat oven to 340°F | Line a 2-lb loaf pan with parchment paper | Food processor

Pour all the ingredients except the dark chocolate and pecans into the food processor and whizz them to a thick mixture | Take out the blade and scrape any excess mixture back into the bowl

Break the dark chocolate and pecans into small pieces and tip them into the bowl | Mix everything together

Pour the mixture into the lined loaf pan and put it in the oven | Bake for 60–65 minutes, or until a skewer inserted into the middle of the loaf comes out clean | Take the pan out of the oven and leave the bread to cool to room temperature | Remove the bread from the pan and cut it into slices to serve

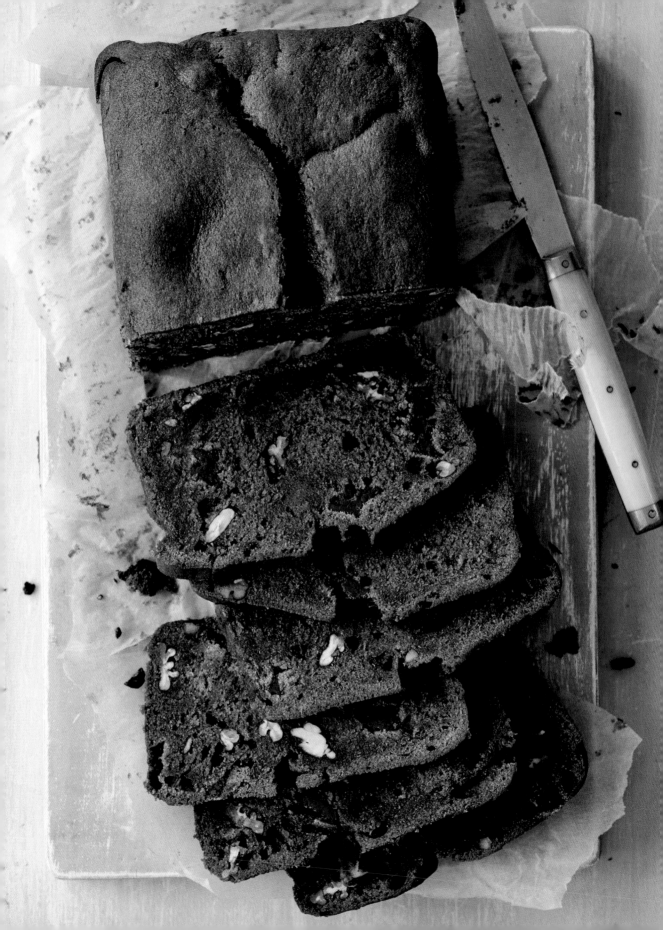

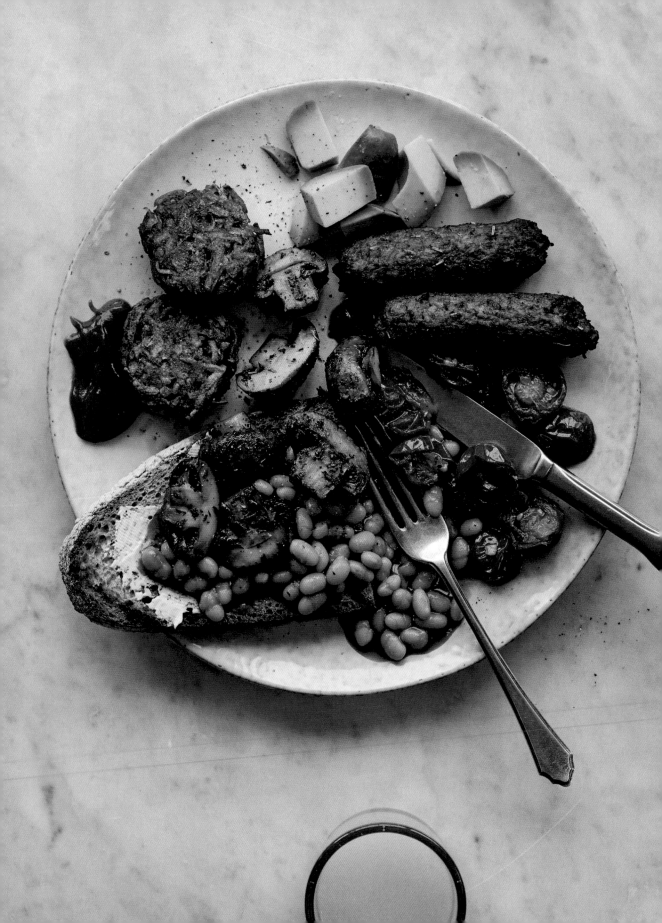

THE BIG BREAKFAST

The only way to deal with a big day ahead is to start with a breakfast of champions. This is a big, filling breakfast that's relatively healthy, best enjoyed with friends. Serve with your sauce of choice and a strong cup of tea or coffee. Feel free to freestyle this one, adding little extras like scrambled tofu (see page 261), hummus, fried potatoes, or fried bread.

(see page 261)

SERVES 2

Hash Browns ingredients (see page 267)
4 frozen vegan sausages
Basil Tomatoes ingredients (see page 266)
Herb Mushrooms ingredients (see page 266)
1½ cups canned baked beans
1 avocado
2 slices bread
dairy-free butter or spread, for spreading
tomato ketchup, to serve
salt and black pepper

Preheat oven to 350°F | Line 2 baking sheets | 2 small saucepans, one with a lid, both over medium heat | Frying pan over medium heat | Toaster or broiler

Timing is everything with this one; follow these instructions and you can't go far wrong

First make the Hash Browns following the instructions on page 267, and put them on a baking sheet | Put the sausages in the same pan as the hash browns | Put the pan in the oven and cook for 20–25 minutes

Make the Basil Tomatoes in the small saucepan with a lid, following the instructions on page 266, and leave them warming over a medium-low heat, stirring occasionally

Make the Herb Mushrooms in the frying pan, following the instructions on page 266, and leave them warming over a medium-low heat, stirring occasionally

Pour the baked beans into the second small saucepan and warm them, stirring occasionally

Halve and carefully pit the avocado by tapping the pit firmly with the heel of a knife so that it lodges in the pit, then twist and remove the pit | Run a spoon around the inside of the skin to scoop out the avocado halves, then slice finely | Sprinkle over a little salt and pepper

Toast the bread and spread with dairy-free butter | Spoon everything on to plates and serve with tomato ketchup

HERB MUSHROOMS

SERVES 2

1 garlic clove
1 sprig fresh rosemary
1 sprig fresh thyme
10 oz mushrooms
2–3 tbsp olive oil
2 tbsp water
salt and black pepper

Frying pan over medium heat

Peel and finely chop the garlic | Remove the leaves from the herbs by running your thumb and forefinger from the top to the base of the stems (the leaves should easily come away), then finely chop | Cut the mushrooms in half

Add the olive oil to the pan and add the garlic, rosemary, and thyme | Stir everything around for about 30 seconds, until the aroma of the garlic has been released

Add the mushrooms and season with salt to taste | Continue to cook for 5 minutes, stirring occasionally, until most of the liquid has reduced down | Pour in the water and fry for another 4 minutes, until the water has evaporated off | Sprinkle with a good pinch of black pepper | Remove from the heat when the mushrooms are nicely brown and caramelized

BASIL TOMATOES

SERVES 2

1 tsp olive oil
5 oz cherry tomatoes
pinch of chili flakes
1 garlic clove
⅔ cup basil leaves
salt and black pepper

Small saucepan with a lid over medium heat

Warm the olive oil in the saucepan | Put the cherry tomatoes in the pan | Add a good pinch each of salt, pepper, and chili flakes | Peel and crush the garlic clove into the pan, put the lid on, turn the heat down to low, and let the tomatoes cook for 12 minutes

Take the lid off the pan, rip up the basil leaves, drop them in the pan, and put the lid back on | Cook for 3–5 minutes longer, until the tomatoes have burst open and stewed down | Serve, spooning any remaining juices over the top as a delicious sauce

HASH BROWNS

SERVES 2–3

2 small russet or other fluffy potatoes
½ small onion
½ sprig fresh rosemary
3 tbsp all-purpose flour
1 tsp paprika
1 tsp onion powder
1 tsp garlic powder
½ tsp salt
½ tsp black pepper
½ tbsp olive oil, plus extra for frying

Preheat oven to 350°F | Line a baking sheet | Clean kitchen towel | Large frying pan over medium-high heat

Coarsely grate the potatoes | Peel and coarsely grate the onion (if you start to cry, give your hands a rinse with cold water) | Put the potato and onion in the middle of the clean kitchen towel, bring the edges of the kitchen towel up, and twist it firmly a few times to squeeze out as much of the liquid as possible | Tip into a large bowl

Strip the rosemary leaves by running your thumb and forefinger from the top to the base of the stem (the leaves should easily come away), chop, and add to the bowl | Add the flour, paprika, onion powder, garlic powder, salt, pepper, and the ½ tablespoon of oil

Mix everything together with your hands until you have a clumpy, thick dough | Divide the mixture into 6 and shape each mound by squeezing it firmly between your hands to make 6 burger-shaped hash browns

Heat some oil in the pan and fry the hash browns for 3 minutes on each side, pushing them down gently with a spatula to help compact them

Transfer the hash browns to the lined baking sheet and put the pan in the oven | Bake for 20–25 minutes, until golden brown and crispy

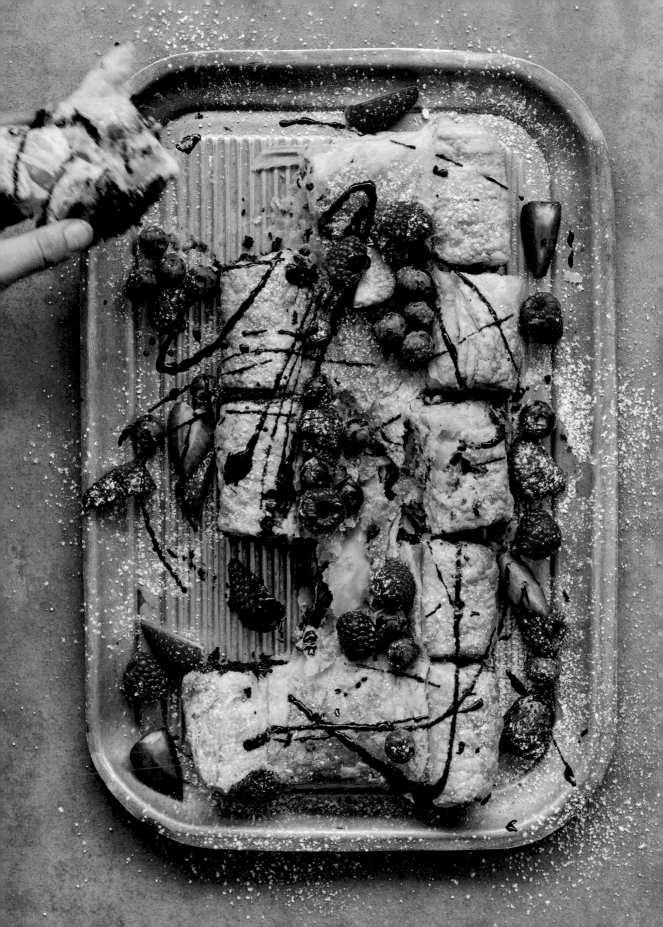

CHOCOLATE CROISSANT TEARER SHARER

This is an easy indulgence, created as a result of our love of pains au chocolat. The store-bought puff pastry sheets make it an effortless, deliciously moreish dish, perfect for the morning after. It's simple to make, impressive to look at (definitely put the fruity bits on top for added wow factor), and just that little bit naughty.

SERVES 4–6

3½ oz dark chocolate
2½ tbsp powdered sugar,
    plus extra for dusting
2 sheets dairy-free puff pastry
2 tbsp unsweetened plant-based milk
handful strawberries
handful blueberries
handful raspberries
oat or soy cream, to serve

Preheat oven to 350°F | Medium saucepan with 1¼ inches water over medium-low heat | Heatproof bowl | Line a large baking sheet with parchment paper | Pastry brush

Put the heatproof bowl on top of the saucepan, making sure the bottom of the bowl isn't touching the water, and reduce the heat to low | Break 2½ oz of the chocolate into the bowl and stir occasionally with a wooden spoon until the chocolate has melted | Pour in the powdered sugar, stir to mix it in completely without any lumps, and take the pan off the heat

Lay 1 sheet of puff pastry on the lined baking sheet | Pour most of the melted chocolate onto the center of the pastry and spread it out, leaving a ¾-inch gap around the edges | Lay the second sheet of pastry flush on top (you may want to ask a friend for help) | Gently press the 2 sheets of pastry together all the way round the edges

With a sharp knife, make 4 evenly spaced cuts into the long edges of the pastry so that they reach about 2 inches in from the edges | You should be left with a strip of pastry running down the middle of the sheet with 5 flaps of pastry either side

Cut the remaining chocolate into 10 chunks and place 1 chunk in the middle of each flap of pastry | Roll the flaps over the chocolate chunks, taking care not to cover the middle section, and press them to seal in the chocolate | Brush all over the top with the plant-based milk | Put the baking sheet in the oven and bake for 30–35 minutes, until the pastry is golden and slightly crispy

Take the baking sheet out of the oven and scatter the fresh berries along the middle section | Drizzle over the remaining melted chocolate | Dust lightly with powdered sugar and serve immediately with a little oat or soy cream on the side for people to pour over if they wish

SIMPLE JAPANESE BREAKFAST

We are huge fans of Japan and Japanese food. A common breakfast in Japan is a smorgasbord of small dishes that often includes miso soup and some rice. Combine these two simple ingredients with the deep umami-flavored sesame cucumbers, and you have a delicious breakfast that can be whipped together really quickly. This will set you up for an awesome day. Turn the page to see it in all its glory!

SERVES 2

Perfectly Boiled Rice (see page 207) or
    1½ cups store-bought precooked
    basmati rice
½ jar pickled ginger
Japanese Pickle (see opposite)
2 envelopes vegetarian miso soup
sesame seeds, for sprinkling
small handful cilantro, to serve
wasabi, to serve
sriracha sauce, to serve

FOR THE SESAME CUCUMBERS
1 large cucumber
1 fresh red chili
¼ cup toasted sesame oil
2 tbsp soy sauce
1 tsp rice vinegar

Small saucepan with a lid over high heat | Chopsticks | Large frying pan

Tip the cooked rice into a mixing bowl, fluff it with a fork, and transfer to a serving bowl

Slice the cucumber in half from top to bottom | Take one half and lay it skin side up on a cutting board | Place a chopstick on either side of the cucumber | Take a sharp knife and cut diagonal slices all the way along the cucumber as finely as you can (the chopsticks will ensure you don't cut all the way through) | Take the chopsticks away and cut the cucumber into 6 equal pieces | Repeat with the other half of the cucumber

Rip the stem from the chili, cut it in half lengthwise, and remove the seeds, if you prefer a milder flavor, and roughly chop

Set the large frying pan over high heat and add the sesame oil | Add the chili to the pan and fry for 90 seconds | Add the soy sauce and rice vinegar | Add the cucumber and fry for 2–3 minutes, until softened but not browned, turning the pieces a couple of times | Remove the cucumber from the pan with a slotted spoon and leave the sauce to bubble for another minute, until slightly thickened

Spoon some rice onto each serving plate | Place a handful of pickled ginger and a tablespoon of Japanese pickle onto each plate | Empty the envelopes of miso soup into 2 mugs or miso soup bowls, pour over freshly boiled water, and stir

Divide the cucumber between the plates and pour some of the cooking liquid over the rice | Sprinkle with some sesame seeds and fresh cilantro and place a dab of wasabi and sriracha on each plate | Serve with the miso soup alongside and enjoy an incredibly easy, healthy, and fresh-feeling start to the day!

JAPANESE PICKLE

You might need to find a Chinese supermarket to get hold of daikon, or you can order it online. This is best after one or two days in the fridge, but you can eat it after a couple of hours. Use as an accompaniment to any Asian-influenced meal.

MAKES 2–3 PINTS

1 large daikon (about 12 oz)
1 tbsp salt
¾-inch piece fresh ginger
½ cup water
½ cup sugar
½ cup rice vinegar
1 tsp ground turmeric

2–3 pint jars with lids | Medium saucepan

First, sterilize your jars and lids by washing them in hot, soapy water and then filling them to the top with boiling water | Drain on a clean kitchen towel until completely dry

Peel the daikon and thinly slice using a mandoline or vegetable peeler (or a very sharp knife) | Put the slices into a colander, sprinkle with the salt, toss to coat, and leave for 30 minutes

Meanwhile, peel the ginger by scraping off the skin with a spoon and cut it into very fine matchsticks

Put the pan over medium heat | Pour in the water and sugar and stir to dissolve the sugar | Bring to a boil | Add the vinegar, turmeric, and ginger | Turn down the heat slightly and leave to simmer for 2–3 minutes | Remove from the heat and leave to cool

Squeeze the daikon with the back of a spoon to remove as much liquid as possible | Divide it between the sterilized jars and pour in the pickling liquid | Put the lids on, put them in the fridge, and leave to pickle away | This can be stored in the fridge for 3 months

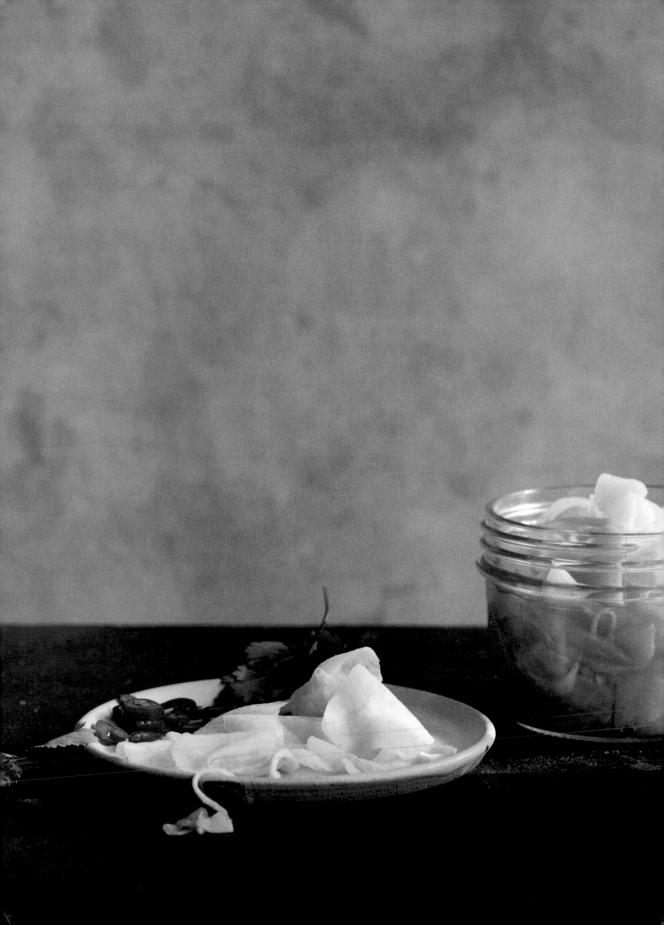

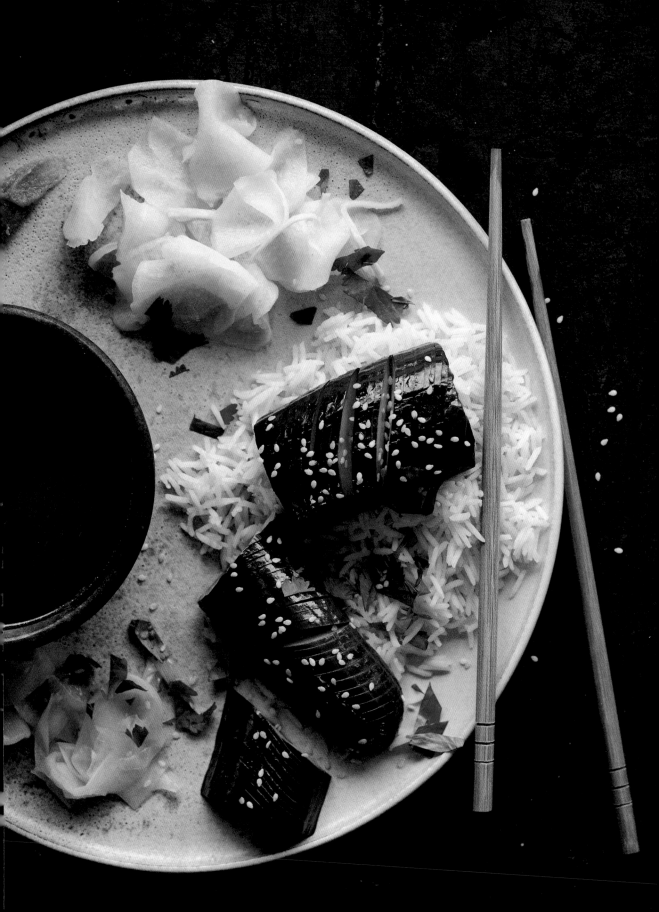

BREAKFAST SMOOTHIES

Putting a load of healthy things in a smoothie is a great way, if not the best way, to start the day. It's quick, easy, and mess free and gives you the feeling that you are already winning the day. These are three of our favorite smoothies.

To make smoothies a part of your daily routine, simply keep a store of fruit and veg in the freezer and blend it up regularly to keep your fruit and veg varied and get a healthy mix of goodness in your body.

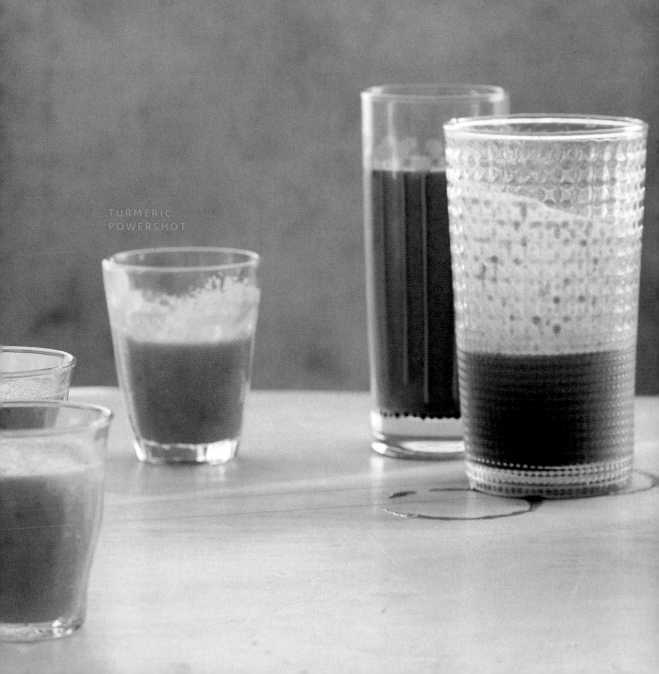

TURMERIC
POWERSHOT

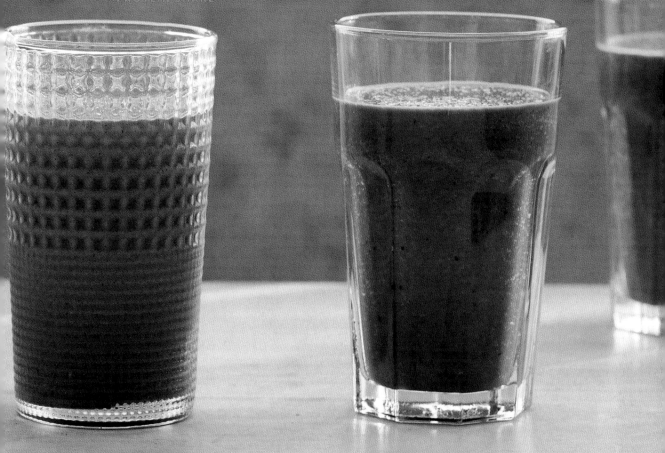
CHOCONANA
PROTEIN SHAKE

GREEN
GOODNESS

TURMERIC POWERSHOT

Be warned, this is one powerful get-you-out-of-bed drink. This will get you and your immune system up with a kick, and gives a noticeable, immediate hit of caffeine-free alertness. It's not for the faint-hearted, but it's very good for you. If you want to turn this into a spicy "Smoochie" cocktail, pour a shot of vodka into each glass.

MAKES 6 SMALL GLASSES

Blender

2 Braeburn apples
2 oranges
1 lemon
2⅓-inch piece fresh ginger
1½ tsp ground turmeric
½ tsp cayenne pepper
7 tbsp water

Core the apples and chop them into pieces | Peel the oranges and lemon and separate the segments | Peel the ginger by scraping off the skin with a spoon and roughly chop | Put all the ingredients into the blender and whizz for a few minutes until you have a thick, liquidy paste

Strain the mixture into a large pitcher through a sieve, pressing out as much of the liquid as possible, and discard the pulp | Pour into glasses and serve

CHOCONANA PROTEIN SHAKE

Who doesn't want to drink a healthy chocolate milkshake for breakfast? This one's choc-full of protein and will give you a great boost for the day ahead.

MAKES 2–4 GLASSES

Blender

2 bananas (fresh or frozen for a cooler smoothie)
¾ cup + 2 tbsp rolled oats
3 tbsp smooth peanut butter
2 tbsp cacao powder
2 tbsp vegan protein powder, optional
1⅔ cups unsweetened plant-based milk
7 tbsp coconut water
1 tsp maple syrup

Put all the ingredients into the blender and whizz to a thick milkshake | Pour into glasses and serve

GREEN GOODNESS

Inspired by Rhonda Patrick's super-green morning smoothie, this is filled with lots of the vitamins and nutrients your body needs to survive and recover. Be warned, this one is health first, taste second, but drink it regularly and you'll feel like a superhero.

SERVES 2

1¾ oz kale
1¾ oz spinach
1¾ oz chard
8 blueberries
1 cup water
½ avocado
½ banana
½ apple
2 cherry tomatoes
1 tbsp peanut butter

Blender

Put the kale, spinach, chard, and blueberries and ¼ cup of the water into a blender and whizz for 1–2 minutes until you have a smooth paste

Scoop the flesh of the avocado half into the blender | Add the banana, apple, cherry tomatoes, peanut butter, and the remaining ¾ cup of water | Blitz until you have a thick and creamy smoothie (if you prefer it a little thinner, add a bit more water) | Drink and feel healthier all day long

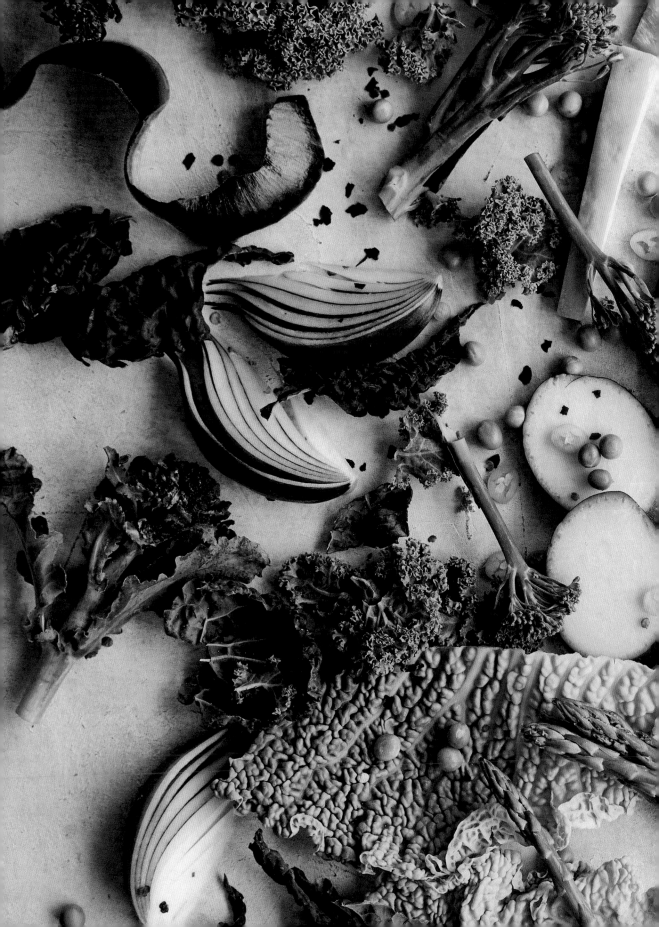

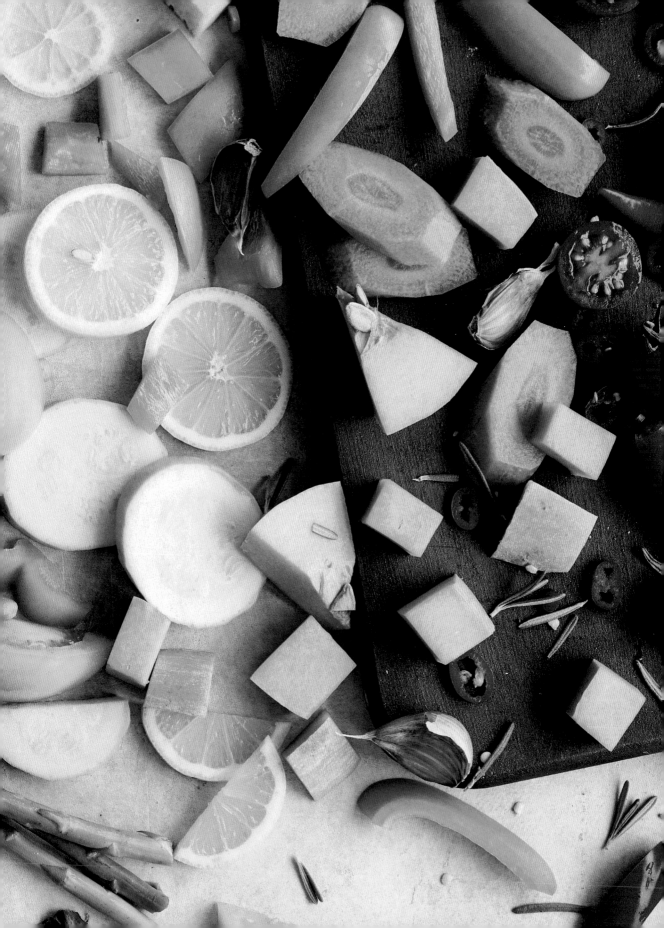

Nutrition

Eating a plant-based, vegan diet is one of the healthiest things you can do for your body. Plus, it feels fantastic. So where do we get our protein from? Plants!

It's a myth that you need animal flesh to get protein. There are world-class athletes who are thriving on a plant-based diet and the strongest animals in the world get their protein from plants. We get ours from nuts and seeds, grains, tofu, beans and peas, and other veggies, both in their natural forms and prepared in things like peanut butter, hummus, and even seitan, a meat substitute made from wheat gluten.

You can get all the essential amino acids from plants, but you do need to eat a variety. Some protein-rich foods, such as amaranth, quinoa, cacao, and hemp, contain all the vital amino acids, just like meat does. But even the plant foods that don't contain all the amino acids can be combined to give you all the essential amino acids. For example, peanut butter on toast or rice and peas are both complete sources of protein. Boom!

In our opinion, a whole food plant-based diet is a really healthy way to live your life. It doesn't include too much oil or refined carbohydrate; however, we operate on an 80/20 principle (thanks, Derek Sarno, for this one) where 80% of the time we eat tasty but healthy food and 20% of the time we treat ourselves.

It's important to realize that we are not simply talking about a typical diet with the meat and dairy removed. We eat a different food pyramid entirely, one that involves loads of delicious fruit, veggies, nuts, seeds, and grains. And if you're eating them in a variety of colors, especially dark green, then you are likely to be getting all the nutrients you need. Opposite you'll find a handy guide on how to get the nutrients that every human needs, be they meat-eater, vegetarian, or vegan.

Good sources of protein

Legumes
- Black beans
- Cannellini beans
- Chickpeas
- Fava beans
- Green beans
- Green peas
- Kidney beans
- Lentils
- Navy beans
- Pinto beans
- Soybeans/Edamame
- Tempeh
- Tofu

Grains
- Brown rice
- Buckwheat
- Bulgur wheat
- Corn
- Oats
- Quinoa
- Seitan
- Soba noodles
- Whole-grain bread

Nuts
- Almond
- Brazil
- Cashew
- Hazelnut
- Macadamia
- Peanuts
- Pecan
- Walnut

Seeds
- Chia
- Flax
- Hemp
- Pumpkin
- Sesame
- Sunflower

Vegetables
- Artichoke
- Asparagus
- Avocado
- Broccoli
- Brussels sprouts
- Corn
- Kale
- Mushrooms
- Potatoes
- Spinach
- Spring greens

Spreads
- Hummus and tahini
- Nut butter

Other
- Dark chocolate
- Goji berries
- Nutritional yeast
- Plant-based cheese
- Spirulina

Calcium

Strengthens bones and teeth, helps blood to clot, aids brain function, and helps muscles to contract.

- Nondairy fortified milks and yogurts
- Tofu
- Almonds
- Brazil nuts
- Chickpeas
- Bok choy
- Curly kale
- Spring greens
- Watercress
- Figs
- Oranges

Vitamin A

Helps your body's immune system to work properly. Aids vision in dim light. Keeps skin and the lining of some parts of the body, such as the nose, healthy.

- Butternut squash
- Cantaloupe
- Carrots and carrot juice
- Kale
- Pumpkin
- Spinach
- Sweet potatoes
- Supplements

Vitamin D

Helps keep bones, teeth, and muscles healthy. Plays an important role in cancer prevention, mental health, and bone protection.

- Fortified cereals, soy products and spreads
- Sunshine! Make sure you get out in the sun for 10 minutes every day
- Supplements, if necessary

Iodine

Important for normal functioning and growth of the body. Plays an important role in the functioning of the thyroid gland.

- Fortified almond, soy, oat, hemp milk
- Kelp, seaweed, nori, and sea vegetables
- Iodine supplements

Magnesium

Essential for hundreds of reactions in your body, such as repairing and regenerating cells and providing energy, so don't be deficient! It's found in chlorophyll (found in green plants), so eat loads of green!

- Avocados
- Chard
- Spinach
- Black beans
- Bananas
- Figs
- Almonds
- Pumpkin seeds
- Dark chocolate

Zinc

Helps regulate and improve functioning of the immune system.

- Leafy green vegetables
- Legumes
- Sprouted seeds and beans
- Nuts
- Seeds
- Oats

Vitamin B12

Helps maintain nerve cells, including those in the brain. It helps your mood, energy, heart, digestion, and more. Vitamin B12 isn't found naturally in plants, but you can get yours from loads of other sources.

- B12 supplements
- Fortified cereals and nondairy milks
- Fortified fruit and vegetable juices
- Nutritional yeast
- Yeast extract (e.g., Marmite or Vegemite)

Iron

Essential for good metabolism, healthy blood flow, and therefore oxygenation of the body. Improves muscle and brain function.

- Artichokes
- Dark green leafy veg
- Sweet potatoes
- Beans
- Chickpeas and tahini
- Green peas
- Lentils
- Cashews
- Pistachios
- Pumpkin, pumpkin seeds, and sesame seeds
- Dried fruit (e.g., dates, figs, prunes, and apricots)
- Tofu
- Dark chocolate

Omega 3

Important for proper brain function and maintaining a healthy cardiovascular system.

- Chia seeds
- Ground flaxseed
- Hemp seeds
- Walnuts and walnut oil
- Flaxseed, canola, and hempseed oils
- Algae-based supplements

Fiber

Helps the body's digestive system, promotes a healthy biome (your gut bacteria), and helps you regulate your weight.

- Baked potato (with skin)
- Beans
- Berries
- Bran cereal
- Brown rice
- Nuts and seeds
- Oatmeal
- Popcorn
- Vegetables (the crunchier the better)
- Whole grains, whole-grain bread, whole-grain pasta etc.

Thanks

First and foremost we would like to thank YOU for reading this book. We hope you love it, and that you find your new favorite recipe in here.

Second and of equal importance, we want to thank every one of our fans. Every single person who has ever watched, shared, liked, or commented on one of our recipes. Thanks so much for being part of the BOSH! journey. We love you all!

We would like to thank Lisa Milton, Rachel Kenny, Louise McGrory, Sarah Hammond, JP, Georgina Green, Darren Shoffren, Ben North, Sophie Calder, Alison Lindsay, Bengono Bessala, and all the great people at HQ and HarperCollins who have embraced us with open arms and embarked on a huge journey with us. Liate Stehlik, Lynn Grady, Cassie Jones, Kaitlin Harri, Anwesha Basu, Kara Zauberman, Tavia Kowalchuk at William Morrow. Whatever you would do, or dream you can, begin it. Boldness has genius, power, and magic in it. Lizzie Mayson, Pip Spence, and Sarah Birks for creating seriously amazing works of art out of our recipes, and for having such a fun month with us along with Steph McLeod, Josh Payne, Clare Gray, Esther Clark, Nicola Roberts, and Amy Stephenson. Paul Palmer-Edwards at Grade for the book design and the patience. Also, Caroline McArthur, Helena Caldon, Jenna Leiter, Katy Gilhooly, and Jordan Bourke. Dr. Rupy Aujla at The Doctor's Kitchen for some badass nutrition tips.

Rachel, Mary, Georgie, Sophie, Blaise, Gemma, Lucy, Avril, and everyone at James Grant for seeing the potential and jumping on board, then helping us grow, grow, and grow. Megan, Becky, and Sarah and all at Carver PR for all their great work, and the fun we've had together!

Cathy, for being a badass with a camera and a machine, a badass cook, and true friend. Bonita, Beverley, and all those who helped out as part of the BOSH! team for bringing such great work to the world and helping us test our recipes again and again and again. Sarah Durber, for your ongoing hustle and ability to help us get shit done. This book is here thanks to your badassness.

Jamie, Paul, Henry, Mitch, Molly, Joe, Stefane, Chris, Bamber, Teej, Lewis, Sami, Chan, Adam, Raman, and every other world-class human at Jungle Creations for supporting us thus far. You guys rock. Pasa, the absolute legend, for all the fun of Pashover and the important introductions you continue to make. Luke Robinson, chef extraordinaire, for being a culinary wizard, an inspiration, and for your help kicking off BOSH! with a bang. Dawn Carr for being a badass. James Heaphy and Oli for finding the time to nail our first few shoots with awesome footage (in between cigarette breaks).

Adam Biddle, for introducing Ian and me to the benefits of plant-based vegan food, the myths surrounding protein, and the wonders of the black. Tim Stillwell at Burrito Kitchen for the giggles. Natalie and everyone at the Good agency for your badass brains. Taimi for your wonderful designs, your incredible work, and your altruistic spirit.

All the people in our world who are striving to make positive changes. There are so many, but for those who have made a difference in our lives: Damien Clarkson and Judy Nadel at Vevolution, Matthew Glover and Jane Land at Veganuary, James Aspey, Serena @vegansofldn, Ellie @kindstateofmind, Robbie and Klaus at @plantbasednews, everyone at Mercy4Animals, PETA, Kate and the whole team at Animal Equality. Harriet Emily for THAT chocolate cake.

Tommy Marshall (Third Person Lurkin), Derek Sarno, Tim Shieff, Grace Regan, Kate Werner, Morgan Masters, Deni Kirkova, Louis Buck, Nicky Johnston, Danny Howells, and Rachel Smith.

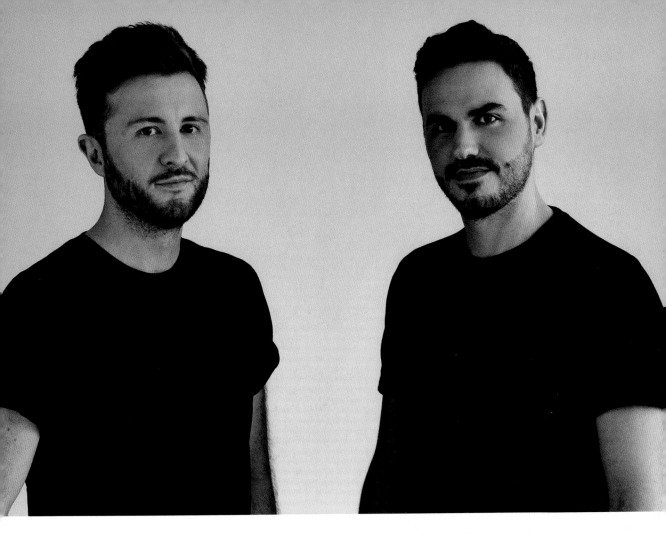

IAN THEASBY

Henry, for your unwavering friendship, insane drive, and faith in me. Mum, Dad, and Frances, for the constant love and support—thank you. Alex, for being there every step of the way. Tom, for being a real level-headed force. Jenny, for your unrivaled and infectious positivity. Kweku, you're a don mega. Joe, for all those late-night chats. Mase, for knowing exactly what the dilly be.

Zulf, your wise words always resonate. CB, for being the ultimate yeah yeah yeah man. Addison, you're one of God's finest. Ben, for being the best rapper alive. Molly, you gave me more drive than you'll ever know. Prosecco Club, stand up! All the London crew for your love and loyalty—you know who you are. And all the Sheffield crew for being there since day one.

HENRY FIRTH

Ian, for your friendship, creativity, work ethic, and patience. Emily-Jane Williams, for being a true worldy and inspiration. Jamie Bolding, for being a hustler, a friend, and a driving force in the world. Jane, Mark, Alice, and Graham for being awesome. Michael, Bruce, Jean, Gus, Arthur, Nick, Sukey, Alison, Curtis, Claire, Nick, and all my family, for their love and support. Kweku, for your expert advice and fun times. Alex for two years on the ship.

Alex and Catherine, for being awesome. Nat and Khairan, for being the coolest people I know. Duncan and Martha plus Ernie, for making me cry. Tim and Susie, for pushing the bunny to the front of Wren's pram. Addison and Claire. Josh, Charlotte, and Leo. Ekow, Claire, and Hugo. Marcus, Ellie, and Jasper. JP, Alex, Anna, Ellie, Taz, Bev, and all the Allplants crew for all the love and support during the early days of BOSH!

INDEX